An Introduction to Psychological Care in Nursing and the Health Professions

D0809431

Caring is at the core of what nurses and other health professionals do. But caring encompasses more than simply looking after people's physical health needs. People requiring any health service will have psychological needs that affect their feelings, thoughts, and behaviour. Good psychological care can even help improve physical health outcomes.

An Introduction to Psychological Care in Nursing and the Health Professions explains and promotes the importance of psychological care for people when they become physically ill, giving a sound theoretical basis to ensure care is evidence-based. It encourages the reader to think about the effects of illness and disability on patients, and to understand what can be done to identify and minimise any difficulties they might be experiencing in these areas. The chapters cover:

- the meaning and elements of care and holistic care;
- a model of psychological care in practice;
- the personal qualities and skills of carers that best underpin psychological care delivery, and how these might be enhanced;
- the knowledge needed for effective psychological caregiving;
- psychological care as it might be practised in a range of health care settings.

This text contains key learning points, practical activities, reflective exercises and case illustrations. It is ideal for student and practising nurses, and health professionals who would like to improve their care for patients in this essential area.

Helena Priest is Senior Lecturer in the School of Psychology at Keele University, UK. She is currently Research Director for the Staffordshire/Keele University Doctorate in Clinical Psychology Training Programme.

An Introduction to Psychological Care in Nursing and the Health Professions

Helena Priest

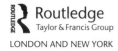

LONDON AND NEW YORK

First published 2012
by Routledge
2 Park Square, Milton Park, Abingdon, Oxon OX14 4RN

Simultaneously published in the USA and Canada
by Routledge
711 Third Avenue, New York, NY 10017

Routledge is an imprint of the Taylor & Francis Group, an informa business

British Library Cataloguing in Publication Data
A catalogue record for this book is available from the British Library

Library of Congress Cataloging in Publication Data
A catalogue record for this book has been requested from The Library of Congress

ISBN: 978–0–415–42907–8 (hbk)
ISBN: 978–0–415–42908–5 (pbk)
ISBN: 978–0–203–80486–5 (ebk)

Typeset in Times
by Keystroke, Station Road, Codsall, Wolverhampton

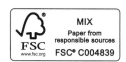

Printed and bound in Great Britain by
TJ International Ltd, Padstow, Cornwall

In memory of my dear mother, Mary Ellen Stanworth, 1913–2007

Contents

Figures and tables

Figures

Tables

Preface

'The development of caring skills must be the primary aim of any programme preparing students for professional registration'

(Royal College of Nursing of the United Kingdom, 2004)

This strong and ambitious statement, in the context of nursing practice, has thrown out a challenge to those involved in healthcare education to explore what is meant by 'caring skills', and how these skills are developed by those entering and remaining in nursing and health care professions. This book sets out to differentiate between the skills needed to care for people's physical health needs, and those needed to care for other aspects of everyday human experience, particularly the psychological needs that affect people's feelings, thoughts and behaviour. In this way, it aims to explain and promote the importance of psychological care for people when they become physically ill and in need of health care services.

Despite increasing evidence from fields such as nursing, medicine and psychology about the centrality of psychological care in illness, it remains a neglected area of clinical research. Indeed, there have been relatively few research studies into the meaning of caring generally. There appears to be little consensus about the precise nature and dimensions of psychological care and how psychological care-giving abilities are acquired. There is also some doubt as to whether such abilities can be taught, or whether they are developed solely through experience, and indeed whether everyone can develop psychological care-giving abilities. This book explores these topics and aims to answer some of these questions.

The idea for the book started many years ago, based on my experiences of teaching and supporting 'general' (adult branch) student nurses from a large teaching hospital, who undertook a statutory three-month placement in a mental health care setting. As well as gaining experience of working with people with mental health needs, these students were to be equipped with some knowledge of human psychological functioning, so that they would be better able to recognise and address the psychological needs of physically ill patients when they returned to practise in adult nursing settings.

These students often arrived with a set of values and priorities which were very different from those whose chosen field was mental health nursing. Their priorities in nursing care were, quite rightly, focused on the relief of physical suffering and on practical, clinical tasks. To them, legitimate work entailed physical activity, being busy, being on the move. They frequently expressed frustration with the nature of mental health nursing work, arguing that in their own care settings they would not have time to spend an hour sitting listening to someone's troubles or observing someone's mood and behaviour, and that even if they did, this would not be seen as 'real work' by the qualified staff on the ward.

Furthermore, they did not see the relevance of learning about psychological concepts and theories in helping them to care for patients' needs. Interestingly, only a few years later, a new curriculum was designed for nurses in the UK (commonly known as 'Project 2000'), which aimed to put a much stronger emphasis on the knowledge base underpinning nursing care delivery. To this end, students from all branches would spend the first eighteen months of their three-year programme developing a firm grounding in behavioural, life and social sciences (UKCC 1989), with very little of that time to be spent in clinical practice settings. As part of this initiative, Project 2000 educational programmes recommended that twenty-two hours be devoted to psychology in the curriculum. My early experiences gained teaching psychology to Project 2000 students again challenged the significance and relevance of behavioural and social science knowledge to the care of people with physical health problems and needs, even when these topics were integrated and applied to practice within the curriculum. It was these experiences that provided the first real motivating factor to undertake the research which led to this book. I quickly came to question the relevance of equipping student nurses with knowledge of psychological concepts, no matter how skilfully applied to nursing. The only reason for doing this, as far as I could see, was if it made any real impact on nursing care. I suspected that it did not. My initial interest, therefore, was in identifying a relationship between what was taught and what happened in practice, and I acknowledge that my expectation that teaching psychology to nurses had little or no influence on care delivery produced an early source of bias that could have impacted on the research. However, Ramprogus's (1995) study of 'Project 2000' students also illustrated deficiencies with this approach emphasising theory and knowledge:

> Students complained that most of the time they had great difficulty relating anything they were taught to nursing. The emphasis particularly on sociology and psychology they felt was more directed at preparing them to be sociologists and psychologists rather than nurses.
>
> (Ramprogus 1995: 86)

The institutions participating in Ramprogus's study claimed to devote between 47 and 167 hours to psychology in the Common Foundation Programme alone, far more than the minimum requirement, but despite this increase in emphasis, students still identified psychology as the most difficult subject to understand and the most difficult to apply to practice, particularly in the early stages of nurse education when exposure to patients was likely to be limited. Owing to frequently large student numbers, psychology was typically taught lecture-style to large groups, with little opportunity for discussion or applied practical work, making it difficult for students to make sense of the material presented to them. This difficulty was compounded when, in accordance with statutory body recommendations, psychology was taught by psychology specialists rather than by nurses, a strategy largely found to be unsuccessful, often requiring nurse educators to repeat sessions in order to clarify and apply information to nursing (Ramprogus 1995).

Many lessons have been learnt from early experiences of Project 2000 courses, and over the years, radical changes have been made to nurse education and preparation for other healthcare professions, such that there is now more of a focus on clinical practice and the acquisition of clinical skills, underpinned by relevant theory and research evidence (e.g. NMC 2010). However, the question of how health care professionals should be prepared to understand and respond to the psychological needs of physically ill people has remained largely unanswered. This question led to a PhD study (Priest 2001) investigating the concepts of 'psychological need' and 'psychological care' as applied to nursing practice, and an exploration of how psychological care-giving abilities are acquired and demonstrated.

It soon became apparent that in order to demonstrate the presence or absence of this particular theory–practice relationship, it would be necessary to identify the tangible aspects of nursing care delivery that would demonstrate that a nurse had indeed drawn upon an internalised concept of psychological care. Herein lay a problem. What did psychological care look like? How would I know when it was taking place? Would I ask the nurse, or the patient, or both, or simply draw inferences from observed behaviour? I realised that despite ten years' experience as a practising mental health nurse, eight years studying psychology to Masters degree level, and (up until the commencement of the study) more than ten years teaching pure and applied psychology to nurses and others, I had difficulty in articulating what psychological care actually meant, and what it looked like. At this point, the aim of the research shifted, and I became motivated by a real desire to understand the nature of the concept and its manifestation in practical nursing care delivery. The search for the essence of psychological care took on a life-force of its own and led to a multi-faceted approach to data generation. I believed that if I could explore the concept from all angles (such as how it is described, explained and used in academic texts, in nursing models and theories, in everyday nursing rhetoric and by nursing regulatory bodies, what it means to practising nurses in everyday caring situations, and how they have come to acquire their understandings), then I might subsequently be in a position to explore the relationship between what is taught and what is delivered. My starting point was my experiences, my beliefs, my expectations; indeed, myself. From this starting point, I was able to reflect upon and produce my own account of psychological care-giving. Another source of bias, perhaps, lay in that I was effectively comparing others' experiences and understandings with a blueprint that I had set myself as being accurate, if not complete. I believe, though, that I was throughout the data analysis and verification process sufficiently open and self-critical to be able to challenge my initial assumptions as required.

This book draws on, updates and extends the findings of this research, illustrating it where appropriate with material from interviews with student and experienced nurses conducted during the course of the research, and from other findings. It considers the relevance of the research findings to the wider caring community, and presents material in a way that is designed to be accessible by and applicable to both beginning practitioners and those who are more experienced.

Using this book

If you are starting out in a health care profession, such as nursing, midwifery, physiotherapy, occupational therapy, radiography, dietetics, medicine, operating department practice, or speech and language therapy, or indeed undertaking any paid or voluntary care work for the first time, then this book will help you to think about the effects of illness and disability on your patients' feelings, thoughts, and behaviour. It will also help you to understand what you can do to identify and minimise any difficulties patients might be experiencing in these areas. It will give you a sound theoretical basis on which to draw to ensure that your care is evidence-based. If you are a more experienced health care professional or carer, it will also help you to reflect on your current practice, consider the ways in which you contribute to the psychological well-being of your patients, and evaluate other possible approaches. In either case, the illustrative material, case studies, reflection points and action points should help you to make links between what you are reading and everyday health care practice situations.

What this book is not

This book is not a general psychology text book, and includes only psychology specific content where it explicitly underpins the knowledge, skills or qualities necessary to deliver effective psychological care to physically ill patients. It is not a book about health psychology, although it does touch on topics often considered part of the remit of health psychology, such as stress and coping. It is not purely an interpersonal or communication skills primer, although key interpersonal skills such as counselling are discussed as they underpin psychological care-giving. The reader is directed to further sources in the reference list to increase knowledge in these areas.

Overview of contents

In Chapter 1, the meaning and the elements of care and caring are discussed. Chapter 2 explores the contributions of psychological knowledge to our understanding of psychological care. Chapter 3 introduces terminology relevant to holistic care and psychological care, and demonstrates why attention to psychological needs is important within the broad framework of holistic care delivery. This leads to an overview and model of psychological care in practice, a consideration of the preconditions for psychological caregiving, and an outline of the consequences of caring in Chapter 4. Chapter 5 discusses the personal qualities of carers that best underpin psychological care delivery, and how these might be enhanced, while Chapter 6 explores the relevant interpersonal skills. Chapters 7 focuses on the knowledge needed for effective psychological caregiving, while Chapter 8 takes a case study approach to explore psychological care as it might be practised in a range of health care settings. The book concludes, in Chapter 9, with a consideration of potential barriers to psychological care, and with a look to the future of psychological care in contemporary health care and educational environments and within developing health care roles.

In summary, the book aims to address the following questions:

- What are psychological needs, and what is psychological care? How can we understand these concepts within the broader context of holistic care in health care settings?
- What factors might activate psychological needs when people become ill and in need of health care services?
- What happens to patients when they receive effective psychological care, and what happens when they do not?
- What are the consequences for carers, of attending (or not) to psychological needs?
- What knowledge, skills and personal qualities are needed? How do carers become able to deliver psychological care in practice?
- What might get in the way of effective psychological care delivery?
- How can we use all this information to improve our practice, and make a difference to the health and well-being of our patients?

The scope of the book

Nurses form the single largest professional group in the health care arena, numbering over half a million practitioners in the UK (NMC 2010), and are the only group of professionals to provide 24-hour 'hands-on' care to their patients. Because of this, recognition of the psychological needs of their patients, and the appropriate response to these identified needs (i.e. psychological care) is largely (but not exclusively) the domain of nurses. Although much of the illustrative material is drawn from nursing, the book acknowledges that contemporary health care is delivered within an inter-professional context. Hence the content is widely applicable to practitioners from a range of professional backgrounds and to the many carers without qualifications who contribute extensively to health and social care delivery across the UK and elsewhere.

Much of the evidence and guidance drawn upon in the book pertains to the National Health Service context as it operates within England. It is acknowledged that NHS services in England, Northern Ireland, Scotland and Wales are managed separately but are similar in most respects; hence references to the NHS and Department of Health can be considered to apply broadly across the four UK countries (NHS 2009). The broad principles are also applicable beyond the confines of the UK.

A note on terminology

Over the years, the terminology used to describe people who access health and social care services (and that includes all of us) has changed. The term 'patient' is often seen as archaic and only relevant in medical settings. Alternative terms such as 'client' have been considered, and this term is still used in some settings, such as counselling and therapy services. At the time of writing, the awkward term 'service user' is preferred in many health care contexts. At the risk of being politically incorrect, this book uses the term 'patient' throughout for consistency, whilst acknowledging that many of the people who access health care would not describe themselves in that way.

Acknowledgements

I would like to thank all the nurses who contributed their stories and experiences so willingly and thus enabled the completion of the research that provided the impetus for this book. Special thanks to them, too, for their quotations which illustrate several of the chapters.

I am also indebted to the people who have contributed case study material for inclusion in Chapter 8: Hannah Firth, Steve Hatton, Helen Jones, Marilyn Owens, Leah Priest, Sue Read, and Karen Vallis, and to the patients and clients who gave permission for their stories to be used.

To my family, friends and colleagues, whom I bored for many years with doubts about completing this project: gracious thanks for your ongoing support and faith in me. Special thanks to my friend and colleague Dr Paula Roberts for her generous assistance with proof reading and for being a 'critical friend' throughout the process of completing this book. Finally, thanks must go to Grace McInnes at Routledge for supporting flexible deadlines, and for continuing to believe that completion of this project was possible, despite many setbacks along the way.

1   The nature of care

Caring is the essence of nursing and the most central and unifying focus for nursing practice.
(Jean Watson 1988)

Introduction

The quotation above is attributable to Dr Jean Watson, and forms part of her theory of nursing. Dr Watson is a distinguished American nurse academic and professor of caring science, who has researched and published widely on the philosophy and theory of human caring and the art and science of caring, particularly as applied to nursing. In this chapter, we explore what is meant by 'caring' and consider whether there is a general concept called 'care', or whether caring differs in a professional context from the way in which we care for, and are cared for by, our family and friends. By summarising some important research and theories of care and caring, this chapter attempts to uncover and explain the key components of caring. This consideration of the meaning of caring will provide the context for the remainder of the book, in which a specific aspect of care (psychological care) is the focus.

What is care?

> **Action point**
>
> Look in any dictionary and see what kinds of definitions are given for the words 'care' and 'caring'.

The Oxford Popular Dictionary has a number of definitions for care, both as a noun, or thing, and as a verb; something that people do. There is no entry for caring. A nursing dictionary does not list either term. If you found any definitions, these are likely to be along the lines of those in Box 1.1, taken from an online dictionary:

Box 1.1 Definitions of care and caring

Care:

Can be a *noun*, meaning the work of providing treatment for or attending to someone or something.

Can be a *verb*, meaning to feel concern or interest.

Caring:

Can be a *noun*, meaning a loving feeling.

Can be a *verb*, meaning to feel and exhibit concern for others.

Source: Wordweb online dictionary and thesaurus. www.wordwebonline.com

---

Within these sample definitions, meanings of care and caring are sufficiently broad as to encompass providing treatment, feeling interested, feeling concerned, and even having loving feelings towards another person or persons. However, there seems to be a world of difference between 'providing treatment for' and having a 'loving feeling for' someone. This illustrates why it might be difficult to define 'care' and 'caring' precisely, both in a general context and when we apply the concept of care to professional health care settings.

In the past 30 or so years, the concept of caring has begun to be given serious attention. There have been several published literature reviews, but until recently, relatively few research studies into the meaning of care and caring. One possible reason is that disciplines such as nursing, which have 'care' as their focus, have for a long time struggled to establish themselves as professional, scientific disciplines, in which concrete concepts that can be studied scientifically through observation and measurement are valued. Concepts such as caring may have been thought 'soft' and therefore inappropriate for scientific study. Nonetheless, in recent years there has been a dramatic increase of interest in the nature of care, caring, and modes of care delivery. This has resulted in an increase in the number of studies setting out to explore caring, an ever-increasing number of theories of caring, and a burgeoning of reports and policy documents in which the concept of care is central. Currently, for example, in England, hospitals and other health care establishments are implementing the 'Essence of Care' strategy (Department of Health 2001, 2003), which aims, amongst other things, to improve the quality of 'the softer aspects of care' such as communication and ensuring privacy and dignity. We consider Essence of Care and its impact on psychological care further in Chapter 9.

Despite this, there is a widespread view that care is such an abstract and elusive concept as to defy description, and perhaps this might always be the case (Paley 2001). Caring is often taken for granted as something that comes naturally, especially for women (Baughan and Smith 2008). Sometimes, however, we are only really aware of what care is when we realise that it is absent, and it is sometimes easier to think about what care really means by thinking of situations that illustrate poor or absent care. Consider the following case illustrations:

Case study 1: Martin's grandmother

In September 1997, Martin Bright, education correspondent for The Independent newspaper, wrote an article headlined 'She was dying for a cuppa. Literally'. He recounted the story of his grandmother who, at the age of 88, had suffered a major cerebro-vascular accident (stroke) from which she had unexpectedly survived, and was transferred to an NHS hospital ward. It was then that her real problems began. Her greatest desire was for a cup of tea, but, it being a weekend, there was no speech therapist available to assess her ability to swallow; without this assessment, no doctor could allow her to have a drink. A series of events ensued over the next few days which Bright variously described as 'shocking', 'a nightmare', and 'torture'. A fellow patient was heard to say: 'It's broken my heart. They won't even go near her. She's been lying there all day and nobody cares'. Eight days after her admission, his grandmother had still not been seen by the speech therapist and had not been allowed to eat or drink (although her nutritional needs were met in other ways). Nursing staff did not appear to feature significantly in her care, the vast majority of which was provided by her relatives. While this patient's needs for physical care and safety were addressed, there was an overriding sense that many of her other needs were never attended to. The result was an overpowering impression of a lack of care by health care professionals, including nurses.

Case study 2: Ellen

Ellen, aged 82, was admitted to hospital for surgical investigation of what was believed to be a malignant tumour. She had until then enjoyed good health and had little experience of the health services. She had been waiting for admission for several months, and it was with great relief that she finally arrived in the ward in a specialist hospital 50 miles away from her home. Naturally, she was anxious about what the investigations might show; about what treatments she might need; and indeed about whether she would recover from her condition. On entering the ward, she was approached by a health care support worker who asked her to wait in the ward lounge, as her bed was not yet ready. There she was to wait for almost two hours until a second health care support worker came to offer her lunch, as the bed was still not available. Neither of these two carers introduced themselves to her, nor explained the delay. Several hours elapsed until the nurse manager finally showed her to her bed. Once again, no introductions or explanations were offered. It was not until Ellen had been in the ward for over seven hours that an individual made human and personal contact with her, introducing himself by name and role, and giving a full explanation of what was to happen during her stay. Interestingly, this individual was a junior doctor, a member of a professional group that is traditionally associated with 'curing' rather than 'caring'. Yet his actions demonstrated greater 'care' than the others whom Ellen had encountered until that point.

Case study 3: Robert

Robert, a fit and healthy middle-aged man, was in hospital for a minor surgical procedure. Upon being visited by his wife on the evening following surgery, his first words were, 'Thank goodness you've come . . . you can help me sit up and use the [urine] bottle'. To which his wife replied, 'Why didn't you call someone?' As soon as these words had been uttered, the answer became apparent. The nurse call bell was hanging neatly in its place on the wall, well out of reach of someone who had that day undergone abdominal surgery, and was still somewhat drowsy and unsteady from the effects of the anaesthetic. An excusable oversight by busy staff? Or evidence again, of thoughtlessness, neglect, and lack of care?

Reflection point

What, if any, deficiencies in care can you identify in each of these stories? Are there any common factors across the stories?

Although in Ellen's case the lack of an available bed was a resource issue perhaps out of staff control, across the case examples, the patients' immediate need was for something other than physical or medical care. Their stories have highlighted how easy it is for patients' needs for comfort, information, reassurance, dignity, and self-esteem to be overlooked. So care seems to be something greater than caring for physical needs, and something which is certainly noticed when it is absent.

Patients' views of caring

To achieve the best possible care, the perceptions and expectations of health care professionals and their patients ought to agree with one another. In the stories above, we might imagine that carers and patients did not see care in the same way. Hence, we need to be aware of the potential for discrepancy, and to understand possible reasons for it, where it exists.

From research evidence, it appears that there is a discrepancy between professionals' and patients' views of caring and the relative weight placed upon particular expressions of caring in practice. Some studies have shown that patients and relatives value highly the more personal aspects of care, sometimes described as the 'expressive' elements of caring, such as openness, attentiveness, listening, and forming a bond with carers. Small acts of caring, such as screening the bed of a dying patient, are viewed as important, and when these details are overlooked, distress is caused to patients and relatives (Philpot 2001). It seems that when care is presented to patients in terms of objective, professional tasks such as checking vital signs (temperature, pulse, and blood pressure, for example) or managing pain, patients sometimes have difficulty interpreting this as 'being cared for' (Paulson 2004). Classic studies of nurses' perceptions of caring such as those of Forrest (1989) and Clarke and Wheeler (1992) (reviewed later in this chapter) show that nurses, too, value expressive elements of caring.

However, many studies point to the opposite (Attree 2001). In such studies, patients are found to place more importance on directly observable caring activities or tasks, sometimes referred to as the 'instrumental' elements of caring, such as dressing a wound or administering medication, than on the less tangible expressive activities such as being listened to or comforted. In sum, there is a continuing debate about whether carers and patients see 'care' as the same thing, and the relative importance each places on the practical, tangible aspects of caring and the expressive, emotional element (Baughan and Smith 2008).

Reflection point

What do you think Martin's grandmother, Ellen and Robert would have said if you had asked them what care they most needed?

Martin's grandmother might have said 'a cup of tea'. Ellen might have said 'information'. Robert might have said 'having the call button to hand'. So perhaps they too preferred practical, easily observed attention to their needs over the more expressive elements of care? Or maybe these were their most urgent priorities, needing to be satisfied before they could even think about a word of kindness, a listening ear, some reassurance, or forming a bond with a carer?

If so, we can understand that at least a minimum level of physical or technical care is required before patients are able to be receptive to the less tangible or expressive aspects of caring (Kyle 1995). This is in line with Maslow's (1954) theory of human motivation, illustrated as a 'hierarchy of human needs' (Figure 1.1), which suggests that until those needs which will ensure survival are met, such as for food, water, and warmth, humans are not motivated to achieve the other needs (all of which Maslow deemed to be psychological in nature) appearing further up the hierarchy.

Another explanation might be that patients do not particularly expect to experience a caring relationship with their nurses or other caregivers; they have primarily come into the health care system to gain help for their physical problems. Their immediate concerns are likely to be getting a diagnosis for their troubling symptoms, or having their pain and discomfort relieved, rather than a meaningful relationship. It may also be that patients hold stereotypical views of their carers, perhaps seeing nurses, for example, as 'angels', and thus they expect expressive caring to be naturally present. Therefore they do not identify it as a particular sign of caring (Kyle 1995). While it may be true that patients neither expect nor want a 'meaningful relationship' with their carers, it cannot be assumed that have no need of expressive caring.

As we shall see, this distinction between carers' and patients' perceptions and expectations of caring has implications for understanding the nature of psychological care, which is perhaps less likely to be delivered through instrumental, observable, tangible actions, and more likely to be delivered through expressive activities.

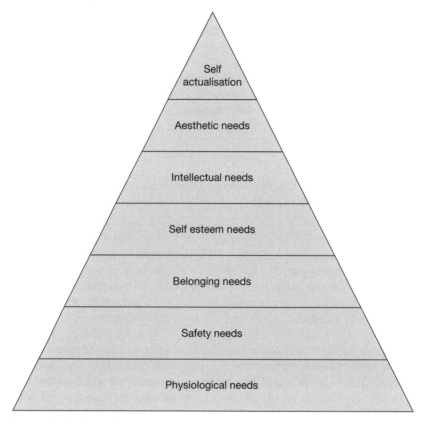

Figure 1.1 Maslow's hierarchy of needs

The relationship between personal and professional caring

Reflection point

Think back to the last time you felt 'cared for' by another person. Who was that person? What exactly did he or she do to make you feel cared for? Can you describe what that experience felt like?

Caring in a lay context

We have all been 'cared for' or been 'taken care of', as babies and dependent infants. As we have grown, we will, in turn, have experienced caring for other people such as friends, partners, and family members, in an everyday or 'lay' context. In your reflections, you may have identified experiences such as when someone went out of their way to help you, or put you first. You may have remembered specific behaviours, such as a hug or having a cup of tea made for you. You may recall feeling valued as a person, or feeling safe, or any number of other emotions. You may have found it difficult to put into words what the experience was like, or even to recall a recent caring experience. This exercise perhaps illustrates how very diverse, uniquely experienced, and elusive the concepts of 'care', 'caring' and 'being cared for' really are, even in an everyday context. How much more difficult, then, to explain what we mean by care and caring as used in the specific context of professional health care?

Many authors have sought to distinguish between caring in the general sense or as practised by 'lay' (non-professional) carers, and professional or formalised caring. It is estimated that there are around six million lay carers in the UK, who 'provide unpaid care by looking after an ill, frail or disabled family member, friend or partner' (Carers UK 2007). Brechin (1999) undertook a study with lay carers of both older people with dementia and adults with intellectual disabilities. She concluded that lay care is 'caring about' someone within the context of a personal relationship, and that it implies an emotional commitment to the person requiring care. 'Caring about' is somehow different from 'caring for'. Although this explanation is not universally accepted, it has contributed to the search for the essential ingredients of caring as it is provided in different contexts.

Kitson (2003) thought that there was a two-way or reciprocal element to caring in a lay context. In such a context, there is likely to be an underpinning close personal relationship, allowing the one being cared for to trust and hand over responsibility to the carer. In return, the carer shows respect for that person's integrity and a continued commitment to that person until independence has been regained. In addition, the carer must possess the appropriate knowledge and skills to meet care needs. Examples of this would be a parent looking after a child with a minor illness, or an adult caring for a frail parent. At the point where the lay carer becomes unable to maintain and demonstrate the required knowledge, skill, or commitment, then assistance from professional carers is likely to be sought. So, for example, the parent might call in the doctor when the child's temperature rose or the cough failed to improve. The adult might be unable to continue caring for the frail parent on a long-term basis due to competing family and work commitments, and might seek respite or permanent residential care for the parent.

In the UK, drawing upon the results of a survey in which nurses provided examples of unique and worthwhile nursing incidents (RCN 1992), Davies (1999) concluded that there were differences between 'caregiving', 'carework' and 'professional care'. *Caregiving*, in Davies's view, refers to the emotionally intense and often exhausting unpaid work occurring in the context of family and friends (in other words, 'lay' caring), while *carework* describes the generally low status work carried out by paid but predominantly untrained people, such as health care support workers. Davies observed that the therapeutic role of such workers and the significance of the relationships that they develop with their patients often goes unacknowledged. This is an important point to consider, when in today's health care climate, so much health care is delivered by people with little or no formal training. So are these 'careworkers' providing a different or lesser quality of care than 'professional carers'?

Caring in a professional context

Professional care, according to Davies (1999), implies that formal knowledge has been acquired through systematic training, and that this knowledge is used to understand a patient's unique circumstances. In other words, we need to be trained to care.

Reflection point

Do you think that professional carers such as nurses need to be trained to care?

Is the ability to care part of the person; in other words, a human trait or quality that is independent of education or training?

Can caring be developed through experience in a caring context such as practising as a nurse?

In later chapters in this book, we will explore the personal qualities, skills, and knowledge that underpin caring, specifically in a professional care context, and the ways in which health care professionals 'become' able to care effectively. Leininger (1981) claimed that professional caring was a different entity from caring in a generic sense, and that care was what distinguished nursing from other professional fields, also implying that caring is a quality or set of behaviours that is somehow acquired through the process of becoming a nurse. Many authors have concluded that professional care is to do with using practical caring tasks to 'care for' another person, and that this is qualitatively different from lay or informal care which is more to do with 'caring about' another person (Brown, Kitson and McKnight 1992, Clifford 1995, Kitson 1987). A further feature of the professional care role is that it involves a contract and payment to carry out the role, and requires the carer to practise within the controls imposed by the health care system (Clifford 1995, Kitson 1987). From these observations, there appear to be clear distinctions between caring as it operates in a personal relationship and how it is expressed in a professional context, based on the presence or absence of a contractual agreement, training, and the organisational context in which care takes place.

Are lay and professional caring so different?

Reflection point

Paulson (2004) noted that 'taking care of patients and caring for patients are not the same'. What do you think is meant by this? Do you agree?

Here we have introduced yet another term, 'taking care of', within the context of professional caring. Paulson suggests that 'taking care of' patients refers to objective, professional care, such as the medical aspects of nursing, and requires training. 'Caring for' patients, however, is a way of interacting with patients that demonstrates sincere care and concern purely because they are human beings (what we have previously referred to as 'caring about'). It requires that carers project an open and warm presence towards their patients. Lack of such genuine care and concern might lead to a patient becoming depressed or anxious at a time when they are, in addition, having to deal with their physical health problems. Paulson suggests that both aspects of care are beneficial to patients in their healing process. This seems to suggest that it is not only possible, but also necessary, to combine the instrumental and expressive elements (or perhaps the professional and lay approaches) of care within everyday nursing practice.

Kitson (2003) argued that the characteristics of commitment, knowledge, skill, and respect for persons, which are inherent within the personal or lay caring role, also form the basis of professional caring relationships. However, due to the contractual nature of the nurse–patient relationship, and the lack of professional carers' personal involvement in their patients' lives, they may not experience the same degree of commitment to their patients. In order to overcome any care deficits that might result from this, professional carers such as nurses must develop a sound knowledge base, a range of interpersonal and technical skills, and respect for the dignity and personal integrity of their patients. Once this has been achieved, the distinctions between lay and professional caring begin to disappear. Indeed, Brown, Kitson, and McKnight (1992) have pointed out a potential danger in distinguishing between the two kinds of caring relationship, because of the undesirable implication that professional care requires distancing oneself physically and socially from patients. Rather, professional care should be viewed as an extension or fulfilment of lay caring. Davies (1999) also believed that professional care carries with it an implicit emotional commitment to patients and the building of a relationship. It may be, then, as suggested by Brechin (1999), that professional care has gone through a long and complex process in order to arrive back at something very like lay care, and that a search for the distinctive features of professional care is no longer necessary. We could, perhaps, conceive of care as being on a continuum with non-professional or lay caring at one end and caring in a professional context at the other (Priest 2010).

One reason for this potential blurring of lay and professional care may be that in recent years, much greater emphasis has been placed upon the psychological aspects of caring, particularly in fields such as nursing. No longer is it nurses' role simply to carry out tasks and duties prescribed by doctors; nurses are instead autonomous practitioners carrying out independent assessments of patients' needs, planning and delivering that care, and evaluating the effectiveness of that care, while being aware of the effects that illness can have upon people's feelings, thoughts, and behaviours. Having assessed, for example, that a patient is anxious about their forthcoming surgery, sad because they are missing their children, or angry because they have received an unwelcome diagnosis or poor prognosis, a psychologically skilled and caring nurse will not ignore these emotions but try to explore and if possible address them. This might be in much the same way as we would try to help a friend feel better if anxious, upset, or frightened.

Caring and nursing

We have spent some time exploring the meaning of care and caring, both in a general or 'lay' sense and in relation to professional health care practice. In relation to nursing, an important question to consider is whether nursing and caring are actually the same thing (that is, can we say that to nurse is to care?), or whether caring is just one component in the broader activity that is nursing. Many researchers and writers believe that nursing and caring are synonymous. The important work and theories of Leininger (1981), for example, strongly suggest that caring is the core concept of nursing and is different from other types of caring outside nursing. Watson's (1979) work, too, suggests that as nursing is the philosophy and science of caring, then nursing *is* caring. Bishop and Scudder (1991, 1997) also, through interpreting nurses' and patients' experiences of care, argued that nursing is the practice of caring, and suggested that the meaning of care and the meaning of nursing are inextricably linked, if not synonymous. Watson (1999) has more recently gone even further to consider caring, or specifically, caring science, as not just the same as nursing, but as *more than* nursing; a concept that unifies nursing.

Boykin and Schoenhofer (1993) were so convinced that nursing and caring were synonymous that they developed a theory of 'nursing as caring'. Their work drew on the ideas of Mayeroff (1971, outlined later in this chapter), who suggested a number of 'caring ingredients'. Their basic premise is that all people are caring, and that our capacity for caring grows throughout our life. Because we are caring, we are directed to know how to behave; that is, caring is at the core of our morals and value systems. In other words, if we see someone in trouble, as a caring person we 'ought' to help them. Because we are caring, we are inclined to see others as caring too.

Reflection point

How far do you agree with Boykin and Schoenhofer that all human beings are essentially caring?

Boykin and Schoenhofer make clear that while people may be essentially caring, not every human *act* is caring. If this were the case, there would be no crimes directed towards other people carried out anywhere in the world, and no neglect of patients' health care needs by carers. We can only speculate about what makes an essentially caring (i.e. good) person do bad things. Psychologists might argue that no-one is either intrinsically good or bad; but that we can all do bad things given the right context or set of circumstances. Psychiatrists might explain that some people have disordered or anti-social personalities, resulting in them having difficulties in forming relationships and caring for other people, a tendency to do only what is of benefit or interest to themselves, no conscience, and little ability to express remorse when doing wrong.

Returning to nursing, there are those who criticise the notion that caring and nursing should be seen as the same thing. Phillips (1993), for example, believes that this has contributed to an over-emphasis on the emotional or expressive aspects of caring that has impeded the image of nursing as a highly skilled practical discipline. It may be that the idea that 'care equals nursing' (and 'nursing equals care') has been influenced by the drive towards professional identity for nurses, one that is distinct from the curing role traditionally associated with doctors (Brechin 1999, Phillips 1993). In other words, care is what nurses do, and is the single thing that distinguishes nurses from other professional groups. We explore this idea further in Chapter 2.

Reflection point

Do you agree that 'care is what nurses do'? Do you think that other professional groups see themselves as caring too?

Action point

Ask a number of colleagues from different health care professions to tell you how they see 'care' in relation to their own profession. Make a note of their responses.

It is likely that if you carried out a quick survey of members of other professional groups involved in health and social care (doctors, physiotherapists, clinical psychologists, and social workers, to name but a few), all would say that caring for others was at the heart of their professional role. With this in mind, perhaps we are left to conclude that although caring lies unquestionably at the heart of nursing's history and practice, we cannot state that caring is the essence of *nursing* until an explicit understanding of professional caring has been achieved. In the following section, we explore some theories about care and some studies that have been conducted, to see how close we are to arriving at a definitive understanding of care in a professional health care context.

Some important research and theory

While there are many theories of nursing, it is interesting to note that some of them do not explicitly mention the words 'care' or 'caring'. The goal for many studies of caring has been to produce a definitive description of the concept and in some cases to detail its essential elements or components. Most studies have taken as their focus the experience of caring either from the perspective of the patient or the carer; with few exceptions most studies have not integrated the two. Here we consider some of the different ways in which caring has been studied; the contribution of a number of authors and studies to our developing understanding of the meaning of care; and to a clearer idea of its component parts.

Ways of studying caring

A variety of methodological approaches has been used to study care and caring, ranging from studies emphasising philosophical understanding and description to those seeking objective and quantifiable measurement of the dimensions of caring.

Philosophical approaches

Philosophical inquiry is an attempt to think clearly and rigorously about difficult topics. It might explore topics that are not normally investigated (or difficult to investigate) in other disciplines, such as truth, values, or mortality. Hence, it is ideally suited to the exploration and understanding of difficult and elusive concepts such as care. Its methods are highly diverse, and in some areas would resemble those followed in scientific disciplines such as mathematics, while in others they would be more similar to methods used in literature and the arts. A disadvantage of this type of work is that 'disagreement and criticism are among the hallmarks of philosophical life . . . it is rare to find two philosophers working in the same area who are in complete agreement with each other' (APA 2000).

Qualitative approaches

Qualitative approaches focus on understanding, describing, and in some cases, explaining aspects of human experience, from the perspective of people having those experiences, in order to understand how humans make sense of their world. Qualitative approaches can have as their focus *people* (such as patients undergoing heart surgery or students undertaking higher education courses) and/or *human phenomena* (such as pain or reassurance) and/or *the process and experience of studying the topic itself* (reflexivity). Typically, qualitative researchers conduct individual or focus group interviews, or observe some aspects of human behaviour and interaction, make detailed notes or record people's words, and try to extract key meanings or themes from the data they have gathered. There are many approaches, including grounded theory, phenomenology, and discourse analysis.

The advantages of using qualitative approaches to studying caring are that they provide rich and detailed data that describes and explains some aspect of human experience. Disadvantages, however, are that because human experiences are unique, it is not possible to generalise to a wider population what is discovered from talking to one individual or a small group of people about their experiences. Furthermore, qualitative research is based largely on the researchers' interpretation of what they have heard or seen; it cannot claim to produce fact or definitive truths.

Quantitative approaches

Quantitative approaches are based on the natural sciences and rely on what can be observed, measured or tested. They seek explanations of cause and effect between variables, and often test predictions or hypotheses. Data collection methods are predetermined, structured, and standardised. They include experiments, surveys, observation schedules, and rating scales. Data analysis methods use measurement and statistical tests to produce numerical data.

A quantitative approach to studying caring might involve using a measurement tool or questionnaire to arrive at numerical scores representing the various elements of caring. Examples of tools that have been used (and in some cases specifically designed) to measure elements of care are the Repertory Grid Technique (Kelly 1955), the Care Q tool (Larson 1987) and the Care Dimensions Inventory (CDI; Watson and Lea 1997). Advantages of such methods are that they can produce considerable amounts of data from large populations; methods are capable of replication by others; and data produced are generalisable to other populations. However, Beck (1999) noted that caring is a concept that is not only difficult to define but also to measure. Thus, in her analysis of eleven quantitative caring instruments, including the CDI and the Care Q, she discovered that although most achieved acceptable reliability levels, different aspects of caring were identified and measured by the available tools, and that they were based on varying definitions of caring.

Theories and studies of caring

All of these approaches have been used by scholars and researchers to try to define and explain what is meant by care and caring, and to identify the components of care. A number of key theories and studies of caring are presented below, to illustrate the range of approaches that have been taken and the various findings.

Mayeroff

At the philosophical end of the continuum, Mayeroff (1971) was one of the first people to attempt an analysis of caring in human relationships. He described caring as a process in which the carer utilised the following qualities:

- knowledge of the cared-for person
- alternating rhythms in the relationship
- patience
- honesty
- trust
- humility
- courage

Leininger

Leininger (1981) carried out pioneering work into caring during her doctoral research, in which she completed an ethnographic study of the Gadsup people of New Guinea. Comparing this group with people from other cultures, she concluded that caring was a universal human trait vital to survival, but that its actual use varied from culture to culture. Out of her understanding that care and beliefs about health and illness were embedded within people's cultural values and worldviews, she developed a *theory of transcultural care*. From her work, she produced a taxonomy of twenty-eight caring constructs, which included both expressive aspects such as 'presence', and instrumental actions such as 'health maintenance acts'.

Watson

Watson (1979, 1988) used qualitative methods based on phenomenology to produce a theory of transpersonal nursing in which she suggested, in a similar vein to Leininger, that care could be divided into two necessary components, instrumental and expressive activities, which should be balanced. Subsequently, prompted by the realisation that the increase of technology and bureaucracy in nursing had led to an emphasis on curing rather than caring, Watson concluded that in order to restore balance between cure and care, caring as a 'moral imperative' was necessary. She identified ten 'carative factors' that combined science and the humanities and which, when taken as a whole, represented a way of being that is a prerequisite of caring. These carative factors placed considerable emphasis upon the expressive elements of care, such as the instillation of faith and hope, but also took into account more instrumental activities such as the provision of an appropriate physical environment. Watson (1999) subsequently emphasised the significance of the 'caring moment' in nursing, in which the nurse creates a space in which connectedness with the patient can occur.

Griffin

Griffin (1983) used philosophical and phenomenological methods to uncover and clarify the components of caring. She concluded that caring was a long-term disposition to act and feel in certain ways, and, in accordance with Leininger (1981) and Watson (1988), that its major components were an activities or actions aspect (the instrumental element) and the attitudes and feelings underlying them (the expressive element). According to Griffin (1983), if a caring activity was carried out without the expression of appropriate emotion and inter-personal attributes, then that activity could not be called caring, although in her view, neither affection for, nor liking of the patient were necessary ingredients of the expressive component of nursing care.

Benner and Wrubel

Through examination of the literature and phenomenological interpretation of 'paradigm cases' in which practising nurses described experiences of caring, Benner and Wrubel (1989) presented caring as a fusion of thinking, feeling and action that was primary to human existence.

Forrest

Forrest's (1989) small-scale but widely cited phenomenological study from Canada claims to have produced definitive descriptions of caring and its elements through the exploration of nurses' views and experiences. Forrest aimed to uncover the meaning of caring from the perspective of the qualified nurse. He interviewed a group of seventeen qualified nurses working in a range of clinical settings including medicine and surgery, posing the question, 'As a nurse, what is caring for you?' He identified key themes falling under the headings of 'What is caring?' and 'What affects caring?'. Within the former theme, caring was described as incorporating the two major elements of involvement, such as 'feeling with and for', and interacting, such as 'touching and holding'. In the second theme, caring was described as being affected by nurses themselves, by their patients, and by nurses' frustrations, coping strategies and sources of support.

Clark and Wheeler

Stimulated by Forrest's (1989) work, Clarke and Wheeler (1992) conducted a phenom-enological study with six qualified nurses in the UK, who were asked to respond to the same initial question as in Forrest's study. Four themes emerged: being supportive; com-municating; pressure; and caring ability. In common with Forrest's discussion of factors affecting caring, Clarke and Wheeler highlighted the categories of 'caring ability' and 'pressure' as an indication of the negative aspects of caring upon nurses, such as tiredness and frustration through not being supported. From these categories, an exhaustive description of caring was produced.

Brown

Brown (1986) asked fifty patients to describe critical incidents in which they felt cared for by a nurse while in hospital for treatment of an acute medical or surgical condition. These critical incidents were analysed thematically in order to identify the process through which the care experience occurred. Eight major care themes emerged, which could be divided equally into those that represent instrumental caring, such as 'assistance with pain', and those that represent expressive caring, such as 'reassuring presence'. Out of these themes, Brown defined care as a four-part process involving: the perception of need by the patient; the recognition of this need by the nurse; action taken to meet this need; and the way in which this action is performed. Brown concluded that patients require their physical care needs (instrumental caring) to be met in a way that both protects and enhances their unique identity (expressive caring).

Chipman

Chipman (1991) interviewed twenty-six self-selected student nurses, and through analysing descriptions of critical incidents of caring and non-caring, sought to answer the question 'what is the meaning and value of caring in the practice of nursing?' Three categories of caring nurse behaviour emerged: giving of self; meeting patients' needs in a timely fashion; and providing comfort measures for patients and families. Non-caring was defined as the opposite of these categories.

Gaut

Gaut (1983) explored caring slogans in the nursing literature and the ordinary use of the term *caring*. She formulated a meaning of caring as comprising awareness and knowledge about the need for care; an intention to act based on that knowledge; and a positive change as a result of caring. In order to care, nurses must show concern and responsibility for providing for their patients. Gaut believed that it was possible to operationalise and measure such caring actions.

Morrison

Morrison (1991) used the Repertory Grid technique (Kelly 1955) to provide a description of caring from the perspective of qualified nurses. Of the constructs that emerged, many related to the personal qualities of the nurse, and many could be described as psychological constructs. Very few constructs related to physical aspects of care. A profile of the ideal caring nurse was produced, which combined a range of positive personal qualities, an approachable and empathic interpersonal approach, and a high level of motivation and concern for others, with a knowledgeable and organised clinical work style and the giving of time. While perhaps weighted towards examples of expressive caring, Morrison's findings confirmed that both expressive and instrumental elements were necessary components of caring.

Lea, Watson, and Deary

Lea *et al.*'s (1998) study is an example of studying caring using quantitative methods. They used the Caring Dimensions Inventory (CDI) devised by Watson and Lea (1997) to arrive at two major dimensions of care: psychosocial aspects and professional and technical aspects. Two minor dimensions related to self-giving were also identified.

Overviews of care and caring

Some authors have adopted a 'concept analysis' framework to explore and explain caring. McCance, McKenna, and Boore (1997), for example, conducted a concept analysis to arrive at four critical attributes of caring: serious attention, concern, providing for, and getting to know the patient. Sadler (1997) also conducted a concept analysis to define professional nurse caring as multi-dimensional work involving presence and a holistic connection to the person in need; this work brought with it both personal satisfaction and a burden.

Others have attempted to pull together a number of study ideas and findings to produce an overview or composite account of caring. For example, Kitson (1993) outlined the historical development of ideas on caring as ranging from 'caring as duty' through 'caring as thera-peutic relationships' to 'caring as an ethical position'. Morse, Solberg, Neander, Bottorff, and Johnson (1990) analysed 35 studies of caring and identified five perspectives: caring as a moral imperative; caring as a human trait; caring as an affect; caring as interpersonal inter-action; and caring as therapeutic intervention requiring knowledge and skill. Nonetheless, they concluded that the amount of available knowledge in relation to caring in nursing remained limited. Several writers have attempted to summarise the 'expressive versus instru-mental' debate. Pepin (1992), for example, suggested that caring comprised the two dimen-sions of 'love' and 'labour'. James (1992) defined care as a blend of organisational and physical tasks with emotional labour. Fletcher (1997) suggested that blending physical and emotional labour into something that can be labelled 'care' is a defining characteristic exclusive to the discipline of nursing. Koldjeski (1990) concluded that both personal qualities (which she labelled as essences) and nursing actions (labelled as entities) should be fused and expressed as being, relating and doing. Ramprogus (1995) summarised the two key dimen-sions as the humanistic aspects of nursing, usually related to informal caring, and the scientific aspects, related to professional caring and demonstrated through knowledge, skills, procedures, and care management activities.

Summary of theories and research about care

We have seen that care has been thought about and studied for many years in a number of different ways. Clearly all of these theories and studies, whatever their methodological stance or precise focus, have contributed greatly to knowledge and understanding of care and caring, mostly with a focus on caring in a nursing context. Common to many of these attempts to uncover and describe dimensions of care and caring is the notion that caring is an interaction between the personal qualities, values and attitudes which enable the carer to perceive and respond to the need for care, and direct, observable action. However, while there is con-siderable agreement about these instrumental-expressive elements, there are some dis-crepancies. There are also those who criticise attempts at reducing care and caring to its components as demonstrated through behaviours, suggesting instead that a more holistic approach should be taken. Phillips (1993: 1555), for example, claimed that 'actions which constitute caring can only be identified by skilled assessment of the situation and not by some universally applicable theories or rules'. We explore the notion of holistic care further in Chapter 3.

Benner (1984), too, warned of the dangers of trying to separate the instrumental and expressive aspects of caring in nursing, and Watson (1988) was aware that the concept of caring could not simply be characterised by certain categories of nursing actions, but was more about those caring ideals that drive nurses' behaviour. In other words, while caring can be revealed by actions, actions alone are not caring. On the other hand, if we do not have clear definitions and descriptions, it might be difficult not only to explain and teach the concept and skill to others, but also to study and explore it further (Clifford 1995). A final factor that appears in several of the theories and explanations of caring in nursing is that it is associated with some personal and emotional cost to the carer.

Conclusion

In this chapter, we set out to explore what is meant by 'care' and 'caring', and have explored theories and ideas emerging predominantly from the professional world of nursing. We have examined the similarities between lay and professional caring, how patients and carers view caring, and whether caring is part of, the same as, or more than nursing. We have reviewed some studies and theories of care and caring and attempted to summarise key components, in order to set the scene for a closer examination of one aspect of care, namely psychological care. In sum, we have discovered that:

- Caring may be destined to remain an elusive concept, permanently and irretrievably (Paley 2001).
- There is a lack of agreement about whether care and caring are the same phenomena in both lay and professional contexts, largely due to the contractual nature of professional care. There does, however, seem to be a trend towards accepting commonalities and a belief that the distinctions are blurring.
- The exact sense in which terms such as care, nursing, nursing care and caring are used is rarely defined, with such terms often used interchangeably. Consequently there is no universal agreement as to whether nursing and caring are synonymous, or separate entities.
- There is some tension between attempts to identify the essential elements or components of care, and the argument that such reduction conflicts with the holistic nature of care.
- Among those who have attempted such a reduction, there is some consensus that both instrumental and expressive elements of caring must be present in order for caring to be recognised and experienced. This consensus is apparent regardless of whether the methodological approach of the study is philosophical, qualitative or quantitative in focus. The majority of studies highlight the significance of expressive over instrumental caring.
- However, when comparisons are made between nurses' and patients' perspectives of care, there is frequently a discrepancy between the two in terms of the relative importance of expressive and instrumental elements.

(Priest 2001)

In Chapter 2, we consider the contribution that psychology has made to our understanding of care, and in Chapter 3 we narrow the focus to the more expressive elements of care, and consider how these elements contribute to our understanding and practice of 'psychological care'.

2　Psychology and care

Psychology does not appear to have made itself known to the broad mass of practising nurses and therapists, and it has achieved little in terms of improved psychological care.

(Keith Nichols 2005)

Introduction

In this chapter, in an attempt to test out and challenge Nichols' statement, we explore the influence of psychology on the development of nursing and health care knowledge and practice. We explore the notion of a 'profession' and how developing a unique body of knowledge and skill contributes to the development of a profession. We take into account the ways in which the professions have drawn on and used psychological knowledge over the past hundred and fifty years, with a focus on the major 'schools' of psychology that have been most influential in health care. We also consider the ways in which psychological knowledge is presented to health care practitioners, through the medium of literature such as text books. The chapter outlines different 'branches' of psychology, and considers how psychological knowledge has contributed to an understanding of the psychological aspects of physical illness, and how such knowledge might help health care professionals to identify and respond to their patients' psychological needs. Illustrations and exercises in this chapter draw mainly on the nursing profession, but key principles are transferable to other groups.

The development of the health care professions

Historically, only three professions were acknowledged: religious ministry, medicine, and law. Today, many occupations would see themselves as professions. We often talk about nursing, physiotherapy, medicine, and so on, as being 'health care professions'; many health care workers in the UK, for example, belong to a 'professional organisation' such as the Royal College of Nursing or the British Psychological Society, and government agencies often refer to 'nursing and allied health professions'. The start of the twenty-first century saw the Health Professions Council (HPC) becoming established in the UK as the regulatory body for many of the professional groups that operate within a health and social care context (excluding nursing and midwifery, which have their own Council). At the time of writing, fourteen professions were included in the HPC: arts therapists, biomedical scientists, chiropodists/podiatrists, clinical scientists, dietitians, occupational therapists, operating department practitioners, orthoptists, paramedics, physiotherapists, practitioner psychologists, prosthetists/orthotists, radiographers, and speech and language therapists. More professions, such as psychotherapy and counselling, are scheduled to join. All of the member professions have at least one professional title that is protected by law, meaning that anyone using any of the titles above must be registered with the HPC (see: http://www.hpc-uk.org/aboutus/).

Characteristics of a profession include having a unique body of specialised knowledge that is not shared with any other professional group; the requirement for members to be trained and licensed to practise their professions; and normally, a set of ethical and behavioural principles that must be followed by members of that profession.

Reflection point: Nursing as a profession

Nursing in the UK requires training and professional registration, and adherence to the code of conduct of its regulatory body, the Nursing and Midwifery Council (NMC). However, does nursing have its own unique body of knowledge?

Is there anything that nurses know and do that other professional groups do not know or do?

The knowledge base of nursing

You may have found it difficult to answer this question, even if you are a nurse. Social workers, physiotherapists, and occupational therapists, for example, all work holistically with individuals and families to improve aspects of their patients' or clients' health and wellbeing. You might have identified 'caring' as something that nurses uniquely do, as in the past, a common saying was 'doctors cure; nurses care'. Traditionally, nurses' roles were to act as doctors' handmaids (as most were female), carrying out the instructions of doctors in the pursuit of a cure for their patients. While critical of doctors, implying that they do not have a caring role, this saying also suggests that caring is central to nursing. We considered the extent to which this is true in Chapter 1, but many of the other professional groups mentioned above would almost certainly describe themselves as caring professions too.

Over the last thirty or so years, there has been considerable development in what might be described as nursing theory, in the desire to create a unique body of knowledge and practice not shared by other professional groups. To this end, the 1980s heralded a burgeoning of 'nursing models', mostly imported into the UK from America, such as Orem's (1995) self-care deficit theory and Roy's (1980) adaptation model. A model developed in and for the UK by Roper, Logan, and Tierney (1980), often referred to as the 'Activities of Daily Living Model', achieved mass popularity and widespread implementation in many care settings in the UK. However, even though later versions of the model underscored the importance of psychological and other needs separate from physiological ones (Marriner Tomey 1998), this model has been criticised as borrowing extensively from the medical model and for emphasising biological over other needs (Aggleton and Chalmers 2000).

Historically, however, before the advent of such theories and models on which to base care delivery and develop practice, nursing traditionally drew upon many other bodies of knowledge, such as those in Figure 2.1. All of these disciplines continue to influence nursing and health care knowledge and practice today. In the remainder of this chapter, we will consider how the last subject on the list, psychology, is relevant to health care professions today; how it has contributed towards the development of these professions; and the role that it plays in helping us to understand the psychological needs of our patients and how to respond to them.

Anatomy (knowing how the human body is structured)
Physiology (understanding how the body works)
Medicine (knowing what can go wrong with the body and how it can be treated)
Law (rules of behaviour established and enforced by the authority or legislation of a community)
Ethics (rules or standards governing the behaviour of an individual or profession)
Philosophy (the systematic investigation of existence and knowledge)
Sociology (the scientific study of the social lives and interactions of people, groups, and societies)
Politics (the process by which decisions and rules are made within a community)
Social policy (a government's means of dealing with social issues and problems)
Art (the expression of imagination or creativity through a variety of media)
Education (the process of acquiring knowledge and skills)
Psychology (the study of the mind and behaviour)

Figure 2.1 Bodies of knowledge that have contributed to nursing knowledge and practice

What is psychology?

According to the actress Maureen Lipman, who in the late 1980s starred memorably as the character Beattie in television advertisements for British Telecom (BT), '[if] you get an "'ology", you're a scientist!' Beattie was, we presume, trying to reassure her grandson Anthony, whose examination results were less than brilliant, but who had passed soci*ology* (the science of society). So, psychology must be the science of the 'psyche'. The closest we can get to defining the psyche is to say it is the 'mind'. Hence, psychology is 'the science (or scientific study) of the mind'. The term 'mind' is problematic in that we cannot see or locate the mind within the human body, so some authors substitute the term 'mental processes' for the word 'mind' – in other words, the activities such as thinking, reasoning and feeling that go on within a person and are related to how that person behaves. Some definitions also include the word 'behaviour', such as 'the science of the mind and human behaviour'. Psychology can also be defined by its aims: it seeks to describe, understand, predict, and (sometimes) modify behaviour.

From these definitions, we can see that while nursing, for example, is about *caring* for individuals, psychology is about *understanding* aspects of individual functioning, so the two would appear to go hand in hand: how can we adequately care for people if we do not first understand them? We could argue that there is little within the discipline of psychology, with its focus on human experience and behaviour, which does not have direct relevance to health care practice. We might, furthermore, agree with the sentiments of Gilbert and Weitz (1949: 9) that 'Nurses have a more urgent need for psychology than have most professional people'.

Reflection point

Is this idea still true today? Do you agree that nurses need psychology more than other professional groups?

If it is indeed true, which parts of the discipline of psychology might be of most relevance to practising nurses, and of most benefit to patients?

Let us start to answer this question by first tracing the history of psychology, and then by examining the contribution that psychology has made over time to describing, understanding, predicting and changing human behaviour.

The history of modern psychology

The roots of modern psychology can variously be traced to religion, to philosophy (especially to the works of the philosophers Socrates, Plato, and Aristotle), and to physiology (especially to the ideas of Hippocrates, who is often referred to as the father of modern medicine). However, some people would claim that psychology only became prominent as a scientific discipline in 1879. Before this time, if it was thought about at all, it was most likely to be thought of as a branch of philosophy. The 1879 date marked the opening of the first psychology laboratory by Wilhelm Wundt in Germany. Wundt used *introspection* to try to understand the structure and content of the human mind. Introspection is a way of looking inward and reporting on or examining one's own thoughts and feelings. We might draw some comparisons between this process and the processes of intuition and reflection which are crucial elements of much professional health care practice (for more on intuition and reflection as personal qualities, see Chapter 5).

At around the same time, in America, William James was also investigating the mind, or 'mental life' through introspection, and deduced that the human mind contained 'feelings, desires, cognition, reasoning and the like' (James 1890). William James was therefore making clear that human mental processes such as thoughts and emotions could and should be studied if a full understanding of human life was to be achieved. From these early beginnings, the development of psychology was rapid, and gave rise to a number of psychological theories and models, most of which are still influential today. A psychological model seeks to identify not a physical or biological explanation for human behaviour, but rather explanations within the person's childhood development and experience, learning experiences, environment, self-concept, thoughts and feelings. Four major psychological explanations of human behaviour exist; these are the psychodynamic model, the behavioural model, the cognitive model, and the humanistic model. We will look at each of these in turn, as well as considering the contribution of Gestalt psychology and the notion of eclecticism (combining ideas and theories in the desire to arrive at the best understanding or explanation).

Psychodynamic theory: Freud and the post-Freudians

This theory has its origins in the late nineteenth and early twentieth century, the major exponents being Freud (1856–1939), Jung (1875–1961), and Adler (1870–1937). Sigmund Freud was born in Freiberg, Moravia (now the Czech Republic), moving to Vienna when he was four years old. He lived there until it was occupied by Germany in 1938; Freud's family were Jewish, so he fled to London, where he died a year later. He trained as a doctor at the University of Vienna medical school but always hoped to specialise in disorders of the brain and nervous system. Freud was one of the first people to challenge the idea that we can gain access to our thoughts and feelings through introspection. This, he argued, is because we only have access to a fraction of what is happening in our mind; many of our mental processes are *unconscious*; that is, we are unaware of them. So, looking inward and trying to examine our own thoughts and feelings is a futile exercise. Despite this, our unconscious mental processes exert a major influence on our everyday lives, experience, and behaviour. Instead of introspecting, Freud argued, people need specialised help and specific techniques to gain access to the content and function of their unconscious minds.

After medical training, Freud opened a private practice for people with 'nervous' disorders, initially using hypnotism to encourage his patients to gain access to and talk about what was in their unconscious mind. Later he used 'free association' (putting his patients in a relaxing position on a couch, encouraging them to say whatever came into their heads, then making interpretations), and interpreting their dreams, to the same ends. He analysed what patients talked about, and the content of their dreams, in terms of traumatic events in their past, and thus explained symptoms such as hysterical paralysis (in which, despite no apparent physical cause, the patient would be unable to move a limb or limbs). In treating someone with such physical symptoms, he might, for example, hypnotise them and demonstrate that in this semi conscious state, they could freely move the supposedly paralysed limb, thus showing that the origin of the problem was psychological rather than physical.

Freud is attributed with introducing the notion of the unconscious mind to the public. He argued that the unconscious mind contains two powerful instincts or forces: *eros*, a creative, positive force, related to love and sexual expression; and *thanatos*, a negative force, linked to death and destruction. In a mentally healthy individual, these forces are in balance, with neither one dominating the other. Some human behaviour can be seen as a result of conflict between these creative and destructive forces within the unconscious. The individual may not be aware of these inner conflicts, due to the operation of defence mechanisms such as repression or denial, which serve to reduce anxiety. For example, someone who has experienced major trauma or abuse in childhood may unconsciously bury all memories of that experience so that the unpleasant memories do not have to be faced and dealt with in adult life. However, when defence mechanisms fail to be effective, the person is likely to experience conflict, anxiety, or depression.

Freud also argued that the human personality develops over the first few years of life, and that initially, instincts are aimed at satisfying all needs. Hence, a child in the first year or two of life needs to be fed, kept warm, comfortable and safe, and cared for; the child is egocentric (focused on itself and its own needs) and cannot take into account the needs of other people. This 'selfish' side of human nature, dominated by the 'pleasure principle' or *id*, persists throughout life. However, as we grow, we learn that we cannot always have exactly what we want when we want it; in some cases, this would mean hurting or upsetting other people or even breaking the law. So we develop a conscience, or a set of moral values, that enables us to reason with ourselves and settle for a reasonable compromise. Freud described this moral conscience as the *superego*. The *ego*, or 'self in reality', balances the opposing needs and demands of the id and the superego, so that in an ideal world, the individual is able to live without excessive stress or anxiety.

Freud was also convinced that the eros, or sexual drive, was a powerful determinant of an individual's make up and behaviour, and was present even in young babies. He argued that childhood experiences were related to specific stages of psycho-sexual development and focused around the part of the body (erogenous zone) that was of prime concern at a particular stage of development. Hence, as they grew, children would pass through the oral stage (related to the mouth and the pleasure experienced from feeding and sucking), the anal stage (related to the rectum and anus and corresponding with pleasure derived from potty training), the genital stage (related to awareness of the genitals), the latency stage (a period of little sexual focus), and the phallic stage (related to the genitals), between birth and adolescence. How the child experienced these stages would determine adult personality and behaviour; any difficulty or 'fixation' at any stage of development would have an adverse and lasting effect on adult life unless treated with an appropriate 'talking' technique or therapy. All of these elements contributed to what is known today as psychodynamic theory.

Freud's ideas, while often shocking to the contemporary society of his day, became nonetheless highly respected and influential, and contributed to the ideas and theories of others such as Jung and Adler. Erikson (1902–1994) developed Freud's ideas of human development occurring in a series of stages, each of which has to be successfully completed before progressing to the next stage of psychological development. If not, the individual would take forward unresolved problems and conflicts that could adversely affect their mental health in later life. For example, the developmental task in adolescence is to establish one's own personal identity as distinct from that of parents, and to find one's own place in adult society. If the key tasks of this stage are not completed satisfactorily, the result may be role confusion or even identity crisis, in which as an adult the individual may find it difficult to establish intimate relationships, to plan for the future, or to channel his or her energies into a meaningful or fulfilling direction. Freud's theories also influenced ideas about child-care, such as those of John Bowlby, who stressed the importance to adult mental health of establishing close relationships through bonding and attachment with a primary caregiver in the first two years of life. Freud's ideas also influenced the development of therapeutic interventions such as counselling, of which we will learn more in the section on humanistic psychology and in later chapters.

Psychodynamic theory in health care practice

Dominant throughout the early part of the twentieth century, Freudian psychodynamic theory exerted considerable influence on medicine and especially psychiatry, advocating that doctors should focus on people's underlying problem rather than the symptoms. 'Talking therapies' such as individual or group psychotherapy, and creative therapies such as art therapy or psychodrama would, it was believed, help to resolve unconscious conflict, particularly in child and mental health care settings, and these approaches continue to be helpful today.

Behaviourism: Pavlov and Skinner

Behaviourist psychology developed from around 1913, and is based on the theories of learning arising largely from the experimental work of Pavlov (1849–1936) and Skinner (1904–1990). Behaviourism challenged not only the ideas of Freud but also the intro-spectionists such as Wundt. The arguments proposed by the behaviourists rejected the notion of internal mental processes, and insisted that psychology should study only behaviour that was directly observable. In this way, internal processes such as thinking, reasoning, and feeling (sometimes described as the 'black box') were seen as unimportant, partly because they were unobservable and therefore could not be verified by other people, and partly because they could be explained as responses to external stimuli which could eventually be explained as behaviour (Hayes 1994). Instead, behaviourists thought that topics worthy of study were human verbal behaviour and specific human behaviours or actions. Behaviourists were using scientific principles to look for connections between actions and events in the environment and the response of the individual to these events (sometimes referred to as stimulus–response psychology).

Behaviourism proposes that all behaviour occurs as a result of learning, and that environmental factors influence this behaviour. Several theories of learning arose out of the work of the behaviourists. Notably, Pavlov's work, known as *classical conditioning*, demonstrated how humans learn as a result of forming new associations between previously unconnected things; in other words, by connecting environmental stimuli and responses to those stimuli. Famously, Pavlov's experimental work with digestive processes in dogs led to the observation that dogs in a laboratory would salivate naturally to the smell or presence of food (a biological response) but less predictably, would also salivate to the sound of a bell ringing, once this had been associated with the arrival of food on enough occasions. Advertising draws on the principles of classical conditioning by linking images of, say, attractive models with sports cars or expensive jewellery.

Skinner took this idea further and looked for how such associations between external stimuli and human responses were formed. In this way, he demonstrated that humans learn as a result of the consequences of their actions. His theory became known as *operant conditioning*, and its principles underpin much of human socialisation. Thus, when behaviour receives positive consequences, or rewards, that behaviour is likely to be repeated. Skinner described this as positive reinforcement. So, when a parent rewards a child with praise or a treat for helping to lay the table, the child may be favourably disposed to help again. Note, however, that this principle applies equally to bad or undesirable behaviours. So the disruptive child in the school classroom who gains the teacher's attention (in an effort to prevent the rest of the class from being disrupted) may repeat the bad behaviour to attract attention on another occasion.

Negative reinforcement is the removal of unpleasant or unwanted consequences of behaviour, and has the same effect of repeating or increasing such behaviours. Thus, when we are in a hot room wearing a warm jumper, removing the jumper leads to a desirable consequence, i.e. feeling cooler, and so in a similar situation in the future we are likely to repeat the behaviour. It is important to distinguish between negative reinforcement and punishment. Punishment is an undesirable consequence of behaviour, and aims to decrease unwanted behaviour rather than increase good or wanted behaviour. In theory, if we are punished for our bad behaviour, we will be less likely to repeat it in future. However, the high rates of recidivism (repeated offences) in the courts and prison system would suggest that the relationship between behaviour and punishment is much more complex.

Social learning theory, first proposed by Albert Bandura (1925–) is an extension of these early theories of learning and behaviour. It suggests that behaviour occurs through observation, and often imitation, of other people's behaviour. In Bandura's famous 'bobo doll' studies, he made a film of a young woman physically attacking an inflatable clown doll (the design of the doll made it bounce back upright when hit). He showed this film to young children and then observed them in their own play time (with access to a similar bobo doll). While it may be expected that the young children would imitate what they had seen an adult doing, what was remarkable in the study was that they readily imitated aggressive behaviour without seeing or expecting any reinforcement or reward. This was a challenge to existing learning theories.

Those people whose behaviour is observed and imitated can be described as role models. It could be argued, for example, that a child brought up in a family environment in which another family member suffers from and displays symptoms and behaviour consistent with anxiety, depression, or schizophrenia might in turn adopt these behaviours and patterns of thinking. Equally, children who are 'fussy eaters' may have observed and imitated the behaviour of parents who are dieting. Many people attribute the existence of a phobia (a severe fear of a specific object or situation) to observing and imitating a fear reaction by a parent confronted with the feared object or situation.

Behaviourism in health care practice

The behaviourist school, dominant until at least the 1950s, was influential for many years in mental health and intellectual disability care settings. If all behaviour is considered to be learned, either by association, consequences, or observation, then it follows that undesirable symptoms or behaviours must be acquired through faulty learning processes. The symptoms or behaviours *are* the problem; therefore, removing the symptoms through a re-learning process should solve the problem. Thus, treatment approaches focus on altering observable behaviours. They include *behaviour therapy*, based on the work of Pavlov, which aims to replace faulty learned associations with alternative, desirable ones; and *behaviour modification*, based on the work of Skinner, which aims to change behaviour by manipulating the consequences of behaviour such as rewards.

Behaviourism has also exerted considerable influence upon the theory and practice of education. Teachers in some subjects today often set behavioural learning objectives for their sessions, such as 'by the end of the session, students will be able to prepare and cook a chicken curry', and go on to assess the extent to which students have achieved these objectives. In health care education, such an approach was used for many years to teach and assess skills acquisition, such as 'students will be able to administer an intra-muscular injection into the correct site using the approved technique'.

Gestalt psychology: Köhler and Lewin

Gestalt psychology, dating from around 1910, expressed the holistic principle that a whole is not merely equal to the sum of its parts, nor is it simply more than the sum of its parts; it is fundamentally different from its parts (Wertheimer 1979). Famously, Köhler (1887–1967) demonstrated that when caged chimpanzees need to solve a problem, such as how to get hold of a bunch of bananas that is out of their reach, they use disparate objects in their environment (such as boxes and sticks, which individually would not help) and put these together in ways that will help them to solve the problem. Köhler claimed that this demonstrated insight learning on the part of the chimps. Gestalt psychology argued that both behaviour *and* experience were legitimate topics of study for psychology. Although it had lost its identity as a major school by the 1920s, one of its followers, Kurt Lewin (1890–1947) used gestalt principles to study motivation and personality, and, notably, small group dynamics.

Gestalt psychology in health care practice

Lewin's group dynamics work and work on leadership became highly influential in many fields; group therapeutic approaches using these principles abounded in mental health care during the 1960s and 1970s, and continue to be used in many areas of mental health nursing practice today. Lewin is said, also, to have influenced Maslow's (1954) theory of motivation and personality (see Chapter One). Gestalt psychology also directly influenced later developments in cognitive psychology and the use of cognitive therapy in treating mental health problems.

Cognitive psychology: Piaget

It was not until the latter half of the twentieth century that new schools of psychology began to emerge, in part due to the work of investigators such as Piaget (1896–1980) who sought to identify the ways in which cognitive functioning developed in childhood. Cognitive psychology considers human thoughts and interpretations of thoughts to be the main determinants of behaviour, and investigates how people acquire, process and store information and their internal mental processes, such as problem solving, memory, learning, and language (in other words, it is interested in how people think, perceive, communicate, remember, and learn).

Drawing heavily on observations of his own children, Piaget concluded that young babies were born with a set of primitive survival reflexes, such as sucking, but soon developed a few simple mental structures called schemas. A *schema* is an idea or plan which helps a child (and also adults when they encounter new people, objects or situations) to work out what things are and what to do with them. The number of schemas we have increases with age and experience, and they become combined by performing operations. In the course of development, a child behaves towards new aspects of the environment by applying already existing schemas. This is known as assimilation. For example, a toddler might have developed a schema for 'car' that is 'something that moves along the road outside my house'. This schema might also include a lorry, or an ambulance. However, when combined with the schema 'something that I get into to go to the shops', the original broad schema no longer fits and needs to be combined with new ones to be able to distinguish a car from an ambulance or a lorry. This process of changing schemas to include new information is known as *accommodation*. Assimilation plus accommodation equals *equilibrium*, and the child is satisfied until a new concept or experience has to be mastered. Piaget described how children pass through a series of stages of cognitive development, using different forms of operations as they grow, to make sense of their world. By early adolescence they have usually developed a sophisticated level of intellectual functioning that allows them to think, process information, reason, problem solve, and make decisions based not only on concrete evidence but also on hypothetical and abstract concepts.

Cognitive psychology developed apace from the 1950s, as did its interest in exploring thinking, perception, reasoning, memory, and information processing. This rapid development was in part due to the growth of computer technology that made it possible to 'model' aspects of human behaviour by means of writing and testing computer programmes. For the first time, it became possible to design programmes that could predict and mimic the ways in which humans might process information, for example during reasoning, problem-solving and decision making. Thus it became possible to begin to explain how these internal processes might operate in human beings. This knowledge added to the existing knowledge of human psychological development, and to knowledge concerning the contents of the 'black box' mediating between external stimuli and behavioural responses.

Cognitive psychology in health care practice

Based on the belief that behaviour is determined by how individuals think about themselves and their world, the cognitive approach to psychology would explain mental health problems as being caused and maintained by errors or biases in thinking. These faulty and often irrational thoughts impair health function, so treatment aims to change faulty or dysfunctional thinking. Treatment approaches include the now well-known cognitive therapy developed by Aaron Beck (1979), more often today combined with behavioural approaches to produce cognitive behaviour therapy (CBT). Other practical applications include how to improve memory or increase the accuracy of decision-making.

Cognitive Behaviour Therapy (CBT)

CBT is an integrated approach that combines two distinct models of explanation and treatment, often more successfully than either cognitive therapy or behaviour therapy alone. Based on research evidence, CBT is today advocated as the treatment of choice for many psychological problems such as depression and anxiety (NICE 2004, 2009). At the time of writing, the UK government was so convinced of the benefits of CBT for a range of mental health problems that it was promoting better access to it (and other psychological therapies) through the Increasing Access to Psychological Therapies (IAPT) agenda, as an alternative or supplement to medication such as anti-depressants.

Humanistic psychology: Maslow and Rogers

A highly significant development, especially for nursing and health care, was the school of humanistic psychology, which was opposed to many of the traditional, scientific and quantitative approaches to understanding human behaviour and experience that had preceded it. The humanistic approach is sometimes described as the 'third force', as it was developed as an alternative to the view that human behaviour is determined either by unconscious forces and early experiences (as in the psychodynamic model) or by external stimuli in the environment (as in the behavioural model). The humanistic explanation, rather, views humans as essentially positive beings with the capacity for free will, for making choices, expressing values and determining their own purpose in life.

The development of humanistic psychology was heavily influenced by May (1909–1994) and Maslow (1908–1970), who were concerned with the meaning of existence, the identity of the individual and the nature of the psychologically healthy person. As we noted in Chapter 1, Maslow (1954) contributed much to our understanding of the notion of psychological need, by concluding that all human needs, other than those physiological and safety needs ensuring physical survival, could be thought of as psychological in nature. According to this theory, human beings are self-motivated to fulfil the lowest level of needs, at least in part, before needs higher up in the hierarchy may be addressed. Thus, physiological and safety needs must first be satisfied. Once this is achieved, humans are motivated to satisfy their love and belonging needs, esteem needs, intellectual needs, aesthetic needs, and the need for self-actualisation. Self-actualisation is the state whereby an individual has become the self that they want to be, but Maslow did allow for the fact that very few people actually achieve this desirable state, as we are usually striving to achieve something more, or become something different or better.

Carl Rogers (1902–1987) is often described as the father of humanistic psychology. Rogers (1970) supported Maslow's view that people have an 'actualising tendency'; a natural motivational force that is directed towards constructive growth. He adopted a non-mechanical, person-centred view of human nature, out of which developed the personal growth movement and the practices of person-centred counselling and encounter groups.

The humanistic model in health care practice

This approach became popular in education, nursing and other interpersonal professions during the 1960s and 1970s, and the counselling movement remains strong today. Mental health problems, according to the humanistic viewpoint, might be explained as the result of people being thwarted in their efforts to grow and self-actualise. This may be due to environmental factors, or not being valued by other people, or being judged adversely by other people. The individual may then develop a negative self-concept, poor self image, and low self esteem, all of which are known to predispose to mental health problems.

Humanistic therapeutic interventions such as person-centred counselling are aimed at increasing the individual's capacity for personal responsibility and choice. The client, rather than the therapist, is seen as the expert; the therapist merely facilitates the individual's progress towards becoming their real self. Counselling skills are discussed further in Chapter 6.

Eclecticism and integrated approaches

There is a view that no single psychological model or explanation of behaviour can be adequate in explaining and addressing the complexities of human behaviour and experience, and that a combination of approaches, from diverse sources, provides the most appropriate 'package' of understanding. This view is known as eclecticism. The eclectic practitioner will draw upon whichever model or group of models of explanation and subsequent treatment seems most appropriate to understand and address individual needs and problems. For example, acknowledging that there is likely to be a complex interplay of causative factors, people with schizophrenia are likely to be treated with a combination of medication, psychological and social interventions, drawing not only on medical and psychological models but acknowledging also that the person's environment and social circumstances can impact upon their health and well being.

Fields of psychological study

The theories and explanations of human behaviour and experience described above have contributed to a number of discrete fields or branches of psychological knowledge and study. Wikipedia lists 22 discrete branches, including specific areas such as 'military psychology' and the 'psychology of religion' (http://en.wikipedia.org/wiki/Category:Branches_of_psychology). Some of these branches share the same name as their associated theory; for example, cognitive psychology is a discrete 'branch' of psychological study. Others are broader and encompass a number of different theoretical approaches; for example, developmental psychology, with its focus on childhood development, would subsume both the psychodynamic theories of Freud and the cognitive development theories of Piaget. We outline key fields of psychology (developmental, social, individual differences), and some areas of applied psychology practice (health psychology, clinical psychology) of relevance to health care in the following section. For more information on applied psychology professions in the UK, see NHS careers (http://www.nhscareers.nhs.uk/details/Default.aspx?Id=446) and Chapter 3 of this book.

Developmental psychology

Developmental psychology focuses on the psychological changes that occur from birth through to (at least) adulthood (some developmental psychologists are also interested in the changes that occur throughout adulthood and into old age). Such changes can include language development, problem solving, moral understanding and behaviour, self-concept and identity formation. Developmental psychology is often interested in exploring the relationship between early experiences and adult behaviour. For example, what might be the impact in later life of young children watching violent TV programmes, or of being separated from members of their family through divorce?

Social psychology

Social psychology focuses on understanding what people do in everyday social settings. The emphasis is on how people interact with one another rather than what they do as individuals. Topics of interest to social psychologists are attitudes and prejudice; interpersonal perception and impression formation; interpersonal relationships; group behaviour; conformity; and conflict and aggressive behaviour. We explore some of these topics further in Chapter 7.

The psychology of individual differences

This branch of psychology is concerned with the ways in which people are different from one another, and in particular how they differ in terms of personality and intelligence.

Psychological knowledge and health care practice

Nursing and other health care professions have, over the years, seen the potential implications of the 'new' discipline of psychology in developing their knowledge and practice and emerging professional status. As we have seen from the historical review, all the major schools of psychology have exerted some influence upon the knowledge base and practical application of health care. One way of exploring this influence further is to see how psychology has been represented within professional practice textbooks. We will consider the example of nursing.

Psychology in nursing textbooks

Most basic nursing textbooks and nursing dictionaries, such as might be purchased by a student nurse, do not define the terms care or caring (Bauer 1990, Radsma 1994), and a survey of general adult nursing textbooks, of the type likely to be regularly consulted or purchased by student nurses, would confirm this (Priest 2001). While such a brief survey cannot do justice to the content of such texts, it does appear that there is scant specific reference or detail regarding psychological need or psychological care. However, these concepts are implicit throughout most texts surveyed, within the notion of holistic care delivery (see Chapter 3). Where psychological issues are specifically discussed, they tend to be restricted to discrete nursing situations such as pre- and post-operative care, or preparing the patient for a physical examination, rather than presented as relevant to the care of all patients with physical health care needs. Thus, although the importance of psychological care is implied throughout these general adult nursing texts, little space is devoted to analysing the nature and effects of such care, nor the skills and knowledge required for its delivery. The novice nurse interested in psychological needs and psychological care would, therefore, have to direct attention elsewhere for more detailed information, and may elect to turn to one of the texts aimed specifically at the integration of psychological concepts into nursing practice.

There is a historical precedence for such material. As long ago as 1924, Saywell produced a handbook for nurses to introduce them to 'the New Psychology' and its relevance to their practice. She acknowledged that the mind is as important as the body and that 'it is becoming widely recognised that it is the *patient* who should be treated, not the disease . . . Good nurses have always recognised this and have endeavoured to minister to the mental as well as the physical state' (Saywell 1924: vii).

It is clear from this quotation that Saywell was aware that physical remedies often depend for their effectiveness upon the personality and skill of the person administering them. Thus, the book aimed to make new knowledge available so that nurses could gain insight into the minds of their patients and give them 'the help without which drugs and operations are often powerless to cure disease' (Saywell 1924: viii). The book was, as might be expected at the time, written from a Freudian psychodynamic perspective, and introduced nurses to the various schools of psychotherapy; the interaction between mind and body and its application to nursing; the concept of the unconscious and mental mechanisms; psycho-neuroses; characteristics of the patient; the personality of the nurse; and nursing children.

Similarly, Wilson (1931), in her textbook on psychology in general nursing, emphasised the psychodynamic approach, and in order to illustrate the mind–body relationship, provided examples of links between physiological symptoms and psychological experiences (such as the link between palpitations and anxiety). Perhaps in early recognition of the theory–practice gap so frequently alluded to today, Wilson provided a chapter detailing ways in which nurses might utilise psychological knowledge in practice, such as suggestion, hypnotism, and persuasion. While most nurses today would rightly shy away from the notion of hypnotism, many would acknowledge the potential to use suggestion and persuasion within their practice.

American texts of the time, perhaps less influenced by European Freudian psychological concepts, offered a broader perspective. Gilbert and Weitz (1949), for example, recognised that the relationship between body and mind was most obvious in a hospital, and concluded that psychology for the nurse was the study of the human individual in sickness and in health. In their textbook, therefore, they introduced fundamental principles of psychology such as thinking, emotion, and personality. A significant part of the text focused on psychological aspects in the care and nursing of infants and young children; older patients; and convalescent and chronically ill patients.

The relevance of psychological knowledge to UK nursing practice was also widely recognised at this time, as evidenced by the publication of the first of many editions of the well-known *Aids to Psychology for Nurses* (McKenzie 1951), later authored by Altschul (1962) and in print for many years. It is likely that UK nurses' interests in aspects of psychology at this time coincided with the publication of national training syllabi, which required that psychological knowledge be taught (General Nursing Council [GNC] 1952, 1962), and were not simply a response to the growing awareness of the significance of the subject matter. Indeed, McGhie, the first of whose many editions of *Psychology as Applied to Nursing* was published in 1959, explicitly linked his textbook content to the psychology component of the GNC nursing syllabus current at the time. He also attempted to provide input on the topics which nurses felt were neglected in psychology texts (McGhie 1979). The 1979 edition of his book covered the four broad subject areas of human development, human motivation, interaction with the environment (covering cognitive psychology topics) and social groups. Altschul's texts covered a similarly broad range of topics; the main differences between the two being that McGhee wrote from the perspective of the psychologist while Altschul's texts had a more overtly nursing focus.

During the later decades of the twentieth century and early twenty-first century, many books have been written aiming to introduce psychology and facilitate its integration into the knowledge base and practice of nursing and health care. There is a growing body of health psychology material, centred on topics of mind–body interaction such as stress and coping, loss, pain, immunology, cancers and psychosomatic illness. Walker *et al.*'s (2007) book, *Psychology for Nurses and the Caring Professions*, for example, covers key psychological concepts such as perception, memory, learning, and social influence, but in addition includes health psychology topics such as pain and stress, health beliefs and managing chronic illness. Upton's (2009) text, *Introducing Psychology for Nurses and Healthcare Professionals,* also covers psychology across the lifespan, the psychology of communication, cognitive psychology, the basis of psychological thought and action, and the psychology of stress and pain. Other texts adopt an explicit focus on psychological skills, designed, for example, to facilitate the development of effective communication, such as Bach and Grant's (2009) *Communication and Interpersonal Skills for Nurses*. Yet others focus on the application of psychological knowledge to health care practice, and a selection of these is reviewed below.

Contemporary textbooks integrating psychology and health care

Despite the growth of such material, a quick search of Amazon's UK website for books with a specifically 'psychological' focus in relation to health care (including nursing) reveals that very few of the 4,000 plus items listed offer an integrated, contemporary approach that focuses primarily on the 'care' aspects of health care. There are a few exceptions: For example, Neil Niven's (2006) book *The Psychology of Nursing Care*, although written by a health psychologist, uses nursing as the organising framework to focus on psychological topics with immediate relevance to nursing, including interpersonal skills, life span development, individual differences, and life events and crises. Gross and Kinnison's (2007) *Psychology for Nurses and Allied Health Professionals* includes key psychological concepts such as attitudes, attributions, personality, conformity, obedience, social behaviour, and life-span development. While it does not explicitly address 'care', it does include one chapter on psychological aspects of illness which outlines Nichols' influential model (see below, and Chapters 3 and 4).

From these contemporary texts, it is possible to gain an overview of psychological topics that are commonly included, and thus infer how psychology continues to influence nursing and health care knowledge and practice. The texts suggest that an underpinning knowledge of psychological concepts is necessary in order for nurses to develop and apply these skilled activities in practice. In sum, health care textbooks with a specific psychological focus begin to shed some light upon the nature and components of psychological care, but differences in focus and emphasis could be obtained depending upon which text practitioners chose (or were recommended) to access. Student health care professionals wishing to understand the nature and practice of psychological care, and whose attention is likely to be drawn to these texts by the fact that students are often the target audience, may be frustrated by the lack of consensus and find difficulty in identifying conclusive statements about the nature of psychological care. In order to arrive at a clear overview of the nature of psychological care and its manifestations in health care, they would need to exercise considerable skill and judgement in the selection of supportive reading material, and are likely also to require assistance and guidance in this selection process.

One notable exception is the book by Nichols (2003) and its forerunner (Nichols 1993), which is aimed specifically at health care professionals and focuses solely on the psychological care of people who are physically ill or injured. It also considers the important issue of the effect on staff of providing psychological care, and steps that must be taken to ensure staff health and well being. This book currently stands alone in the UK in this respect, and Nichols' frameworks for psychological care are presented and discussed further in Chapters 3 and 4.

Summary

This chapter has traced the development of psychological knowledge and its impact upon health care practice through significant theories developed over the past hundred or so years. It has also considered how such knowledge is translated to the health care professions through the medium of textbooks. Returning to Nichols' statement that opened this chapter, we may now be in a better position to judge whether psychology has, in fact, made itself known to the broad mass of practising nurses and therapists, and whether it has achieved anything in terms of improved psychological care. In Chapter 3, we begin to explore the ways in which 'psychology' and 'care' can come together in addressing the psychological needs of physically ill patients.

3 Psychological needs in illness

Symptoms . . . are very often not symptoms of the disease at all, but of something quite different . . .

(Florence Nightingale 1859)

Introduction

In Chapter 1, we looked at the nature of caring, both in general terms and specifically in relation to professional practice. The chapter concluded with an attempt to pull 'caring' apart; that is, to identify its key components and characteristics. In Chapter 2, we began to trace the contribution that the discipline of psychology has made to health care practice and to our understanding of the 'psychological' component of care delivery.

Leading directly from these chapters, this chapter begins to demonstrate how psychology and health care can come together, through a focus on psychological needs and psychological care. Although the term 'psychological care' is commonplace in health care settings, there is frequently little or no explanation of what it means, nor how such care is to be delivered. This chapter will introduce relevant terminology within the broad framework of what might be described as holistic care. Drawing upon research evidence, we consider why it is important to identify and care for the psychological needs of people who are ill, and the challenges of doing so. We also review the interface between psychological needs and psychological or mental health problems. The chapter will also consider the contributions of a range of specialist professions including health psychology, clinical psychology and psychiatry, in aiding our understanding of and responses to these needs, and explore the roles of some of these specialist workers.

Care and psychological care

As we saw in Chapter 1, there has been a considerable amount of research carried out aimed at understanding the meaning of 'care' and 'caring' in health care practice, and a number of theories of care have been developed over the past thirty or so years. Additionally, UK health care practice, and particularly nursing, has been heavily influenced by a number of models and theories, many imported from the USA (for example, Orem's [1995] self-care deficit theory and Roy's [1980] adaptation model), and often not entirely applicable within UK settings. Critiques of these models (e.g. Fraser 1996; Phillips *et al.* 1998), however, suggest that they have not been particularly helpful in guiding nurses towards identifying and responding to psychological needs.

In sum, the part of caring that is about looking after patients' psychological needs, although implicit within caring theories and within nursing models and theories, has not been well studied. There is scarce and sometimes conflicting evidence available about the nature and delivery of skilled psychological care and of the processes involved in becoming an effective psychological caregiver. We have seen that caring is a broad and pervasive concept that perhaps defies definition, and we might imagine that the 'psychological' part of care is closely aligned with the expressive aspect of caring. If this is the case, then psychological care is not only a necessary element of caring but also a significant one.

While it may be difficult to arrive at a complete consensus on the nature and meaning of psychological care, that should not prevent us from trying to understand it, consider its place within effective care delivery, and think about how we can develop the necessary knowledge, skills, and personal qualities in a relevant and effective way. To set the exploration of psychological care in context, we will look more closely at the concept of *holism* and how it is relevant to professional health care.

Holism and health care

The word holism derives from the Greek holos, meaning whole, and the over-riding principle of holism is that the 'whole' of anything is more than the sum of its parts. Furthermore, the parts must be integrated in order to achieve harmony, and any change or disturbance in one part creates change or disruption in the whole.

Principles of holism: a practical illustration

A simple example might make these principles clear. Imagine that you have purchased a piece of self-assembly furniture, say, a coffee table. You empty the contents of the box onto the floor and check that you do indeed have all the parts required to construct the table. However, despite having all the parts, you do not have a table until you have assembled them in the correct way and in the correct order. The finished product is therefore more than a collection of its individual components. Now imagine that a key component is faulty (one leg is the wrong length, for example). You can still assemble the table, following the instructions, and no parts are missing. But do you still have a table? Or do you have something that looks a little like a table but is so wobbly that it cannot be used to rest your cup on without it sliding off and spilling your coffee on the floor? In this way, we can see that if one part of the table is not working correctly, this will cause the whole table to malfunction.

Reflection point

How well do you think the concept of holism applies to human beings?
Are human beings always seen as 'whole'?
   Can you think of an example where they are seen instead as a collection of separate parts?

Holism can also be defined in terms of its opposite, which is reductionism. Reductionism seeks to understand things by breaking them down into their component parts. Modern medicine is sometimes considered reductionist in its approach, since it is organised according to specialities relating to parts of the human body, or aspects of human functioning. Hence, a dermatologist will treat skin problems; an orthopaedic surgeon will treat bone and joint problems, and so on. This does not, of course, imply that specialist doctors only see the patient's skin or broken bone, and discount the 'person' with the problem; good modern medicine considers all aspects of an individual patient's functioning and lifestyle in assessing needs, arriving at diagnoses, and prescribing treatment.

Although the term 'holism' was not introduced until 1926 by Smuts, a South African philosopher, the origins of the concept can be traced back at least as far as Hippocrates, who is thought of as the father of modern medicine. Writing in the fifth century BC, Hippocrates emphasised the importance of environmental, emotional, and nutritional factors in illness and treatment. Such ideas are intrinsic to Eastern healing traditions. For example, traditional Indian Ayurveda is a philosophy and system of healing the whole person, both body and mind. The origins of this system go back to the distant past, in which philosophy and medicine were not separate disciplines, as they are today. Ayurvedic healing addresses broad elements of an individual's lifestyle such as spiritual life, diet, and exercise, and prescribes remedies such as yoga, herbal therapy, and massage.

Similarly, the Chinese healing tradition focuses on the Tao (see Figure 3.1).

Within the Tao, health is represented as a balance between an individual's 'female' or Yin characteristics, such as being inward-looking, cold, negative, passive, and receptive, and the 'male' or Yang characteristics such as being outward-looking, hot, positive, active, and creative. Chinese healing encompasses techniques such as meditation, exercise, diet, manual manipulative techniques, burning herbs, acupuncture, and herbal medicines, and it is of note that Chinese medicine shops are frequently found today within Western shopping centres offering consultation, advice and treatment on a range of health problems such as skin and allergic disorders.

In the Western world, a broad notion of health underpinned the ideas of Florence Nightingale (1820–1910), widely considered to be the founder of modern nursing practice and education in the UK and elsewhere. She was acutely aware that what might appear to be a physical illness or symptom in an individual could equally be attributed to other factors, such as poor hygiene, and she emphasised the importance of elements such as cleanliness, diet, and light in improving health. These factors suggest discomfort or 'dis-ease', as much as illness/disease. We might therefore conclude that they are necessary components of care,

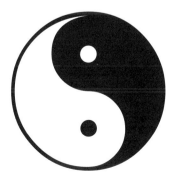

Figure 3.1 Tao symbol

without which patients' recovery from illness will be hindered. So, Florence Nightingale was clear that good health required more than attention to physical needs, and could therefore be described as a holistic practitioner and theorist. Her ideas were captured in an early World Health Organisation (WHO) definition of health as 'a state of complete physical, mental and social well-being and not merely the absence of disease or infirmity' (WHO 1946). In this way, we can see health as synonymous with wholeness.

If holism implies wholeness and balance, then holistic care, in a health context, can be seen as a balance in meeting all of a patient's needs.

Action point

What do you think are the 'parts' that go to make up a whole person?

There are many ways of answering this question, but writers often refer to humans as having 'bio-psycho-social' components – in other words, a body (bio), a soul or mind (psycho), and a social world in which they live in relation to other people (Sarafino 2005; Alladdin 2009). Some writers further subdivide the 'social' component into cultural aspects, which might include racial and ethnic identity, and environmental aspects, which might include the area in which the person lives, or the quality of their housing. Yet others add in a spiritual dimension – a sense of being connected to something greater than oneself, which is sometimes expressed as a religious belief.

In recent years, health care professions have begun to embrace holism as the foundation of health and health care. In 1980, for example, the American Holistic Nurses' Association (AHNA) was founded to renew and enhance the art of caring for the whole person. The organisation embraces nursing as both a lifestyle and a profession, and believes that because true healing comes from within, nurses must first heal themselves before they can facilitate the healing of others. Similarly, in the UK, the British Holistic Medical Association (BHMA) was founded in 1983, with the aim of educating doctors, medical students, allied health professionals, and members of the general public in the principles and practice of holistic medicine. The BHMA (2010) believes that while using technologies to remedy biological faults is of immense value, health care cannot be based on the body alone. Effective, humane health care must take into account people's thoughts and feelings, their relationships and spiritual life. As with the AHNA, the BHMA believes that those who work in health care must understand and take care of their own needs as well as the needs of those they look after.

These recent developments are encouraging, but given that Florence Nightingale was considered to be the first holistic nurse (AHNA 2010), it is surprising perhaps that it is only in the past thirty years that there has been a major renewal of interest in the concept from health care practitioners worldwide.

Reflection point

Could the health care professions, at some time, have lost the art of caring for the whole person? If so, why might this have happened?

What might have happened to holism between Florence Nightingale's time and the 1980s?

Although holism remains central to the principles of many Eastern healing traditions, it seems that the domination of Western health care by technological and medical advances during the twentieth century diminished the significance of non-medical contributions to health care. Such advances include greater knowledge of human anatomy and physiology; technical developments (such as surgical procedures, equipment such as x-ray machines and scanners, drugs, and information technology); the dominance of science and technology in health care; and the emergence and pre-eminence of the 'medical model'. These developments have perhaps resulted in a primary focus on the body and physical functioning, and less on the psychological and social aspects of human functioning.

The medical model

The medical model describes an approach to health care and treatment that was dominant in the Western world until the latter part of the twentieth century. René Descartes (1596–1650), a French philosopher, mathematician, scientist and writer, believed that the mind and the body were separate entities, with the body being a complex machine, and the mind being the home of the 'soul'. These ideas, sometimes referred to as Cartesian dualism (from Descartes' name and from the idea that the mind and body are two separate things [dualism]), influenced scientific thinking and practice for centuries, and certainly informed modern medicine. In the medical model, ideas of health centre on the physical body, and health is largely defined in negative terms; thus, symptoms need to be eliminated, and illnesses need to be cured or removed. The doctor is the expert who prescribes medical treatment; other members of the health care team carry it out. The patient need not be actively involved. A 'tongue in cheek' view of the medical model and its aims is provided by Ragins (2002): 'A comfortable treatment relationship between powerful healing professionals and helpless patients complying with orders they need not really understand results in a clear recovery'.

Such an extreme view of the medical model is rightly challenged nowadays, in part because most medical practitioners do not see themselves as 'powerful healing professionals' who exclude their patients from their own care and treatment. Equally, the growing influence and success of ideas from other cultures and other professional groups has contributed to a more comprehensive remit for modern medicine. Furthermore, an increasing awareness that the mind and body are not so separate, as Descartes proposed, has contributed to changing views.

For example, there are many apparently physical illnesses, such as migraine, asthma, and some skin conditions, that are triggered or made more severe if the sufferer is under emotional stress. These conditions are sometimes described as psychosomatic disorders, to demonstrate the interrelationship between a person's *psyche* (the Greek word for human soul or personality; sometimes translated as 'mind') and *soma* (the Greek word for body). We are becoming increasingly aware that stress can have an adverse effect on the body's immune system, which instead of protecting the individual against illness, actually reduces people's physical defence against illness, and predisposes them to develop viral conditions (such as colds and sore throats) or more serious problems, such as cancer. Equally, we are becoming aware of a wide range of illnesses which do not have a demonstrable physical cause, such as Myalgic Encephalitis/Chronic Fatigue Syndrome (ME/CFS), but which are undoubtedly illnesses and cause a great deal of physical suffering. However, it is important to note that although we are increasingly recognising that the body and mind are intimately connected, we are not rejecting the medical model outright. Instead, a more holistic approach tries to complement medical, technical, and scientific precision with techniques from other sources, times or cultures, and thus to address the whole person rather than a single aspect of the person's physical functioning. Hence, the traditional 'medical model' approach has largely been superseded by the understanding that the mind and body are not so separate, and that a holistic approach is more appropriate (Federoff and Gostin 2009). Despite this, it is often thought that 'the dualistic notions of biomedicine still dominate contemporary health care, despite evidence of the limitations' (Harrison 2001: 48).

How does the concept of holism translate into everyday health care practice? The concept can be viewed as a *philosophy* or world view, or as a *practical tool* for care delivery, or as a combination of the two. As a philosophy, holism is an ideal, a view of the person as a holistic being. Health and wellness are seen as the goals of holism, and a desire to see the individual as a whole person at all times will underpin all caring practices and activities. In the words of the AHNA (2010), holistic nursing is 'not necessarily something that you do: it is an attitude, a philosophy, and a way of being'. In contrast, holism can also be seen as having a more practical application; one in which the carer's activities help the patient in his or her journey towards health care, or assist with recovery, or aid transition to peaceful death. In relation to nursing, holistic nursing has been described as 'the desire to respond sensitively to the reality of the other . . . from an empathic viewpoint' (Warelow 1996: 657). We will explore what is meant by having an 'empathic viewpoint' further in Chapter Five. For now, the fundamental message is that in delivering holistic care, patients should be viewed as more than and different from the sum of their parts, and certainly as more than their physical bodies. In delivering care, we must therefore consider all activities affecting every aspect of the patient's life, and recognise and respond to the wholeness of the individual.

Reflection point

- Thinking about your current or recent clinical experiences, identify one element of your practice that you consider to be holistic.
- Describe this practice, identifying the features that make it holistic.
- Identify factors that might prevent this practice from being carried out.

Barriers to holistic care

Although there is evidence that the philosophy of holistic care has been widely discussed and accepted, there is often difficulty in translating the concept into a practical tool for care delivery, particularly in general adult care settings (McMahon 1991; Henderson 2002). This may be due to a lack of clarity in the meaning of the concept or to a lack of practical guidelines. Henderson showed that nurses have difficulty in translating theoretical knowledge about holistic care that they have learnt in the classroom into practice, in part because of a perceived expectation that they should be competing practical tasks. A further difficulty is the tension between reductionist and holistic approaches within health care. Because of the way in which western health care systems and medicine are organised, according to specialities corresponding with parts of a person's body or particular aspects of function, it is almost impossible to avoid reductionism in health care; thus strategies have to be found in which holistic approaches can be complementary to reductionism.

Further challenges face carers who wish to provide holistic care. First, it is unlikely that any one individual can fully meet the needs of another, therefore co-operation and effective teamwork are required. Second, if the concept is taken to its extreme, we might have difficulty identifying the boundaries of our practice, and find ourselves encompassing roles that would normally be undertaken by others. Being unable to provide total care would undoubtedly lead to role strain and conflict, emotional stress and burnout. This, in turn, may lead to a lack of care or in tasks being carried out in a reluctant manner. The concept of 'emotional labour' (James 1989; Smith and Gray 2001), long recognised in nursing, occurs where nurses 'manage' their strong and often conflicting emotions, suppressing them where necessary, to give an outward appearance of being caring to their patients and thus able to survive in the emotionally demanding world of nursing practice. It is likely that this concept applies also to other health care professions. We will explore the concept of emotional labour further in Chapter 9.

Given these difficulties, in reality often only token attention is paid to the concept of holistic care. In fact, some would say that attempts to deal simultaneously with the physical, psychological, and social needs of patients may be impossible, rendering the application of holism to practice unachievable, and leading to the conclusion that 'it may usefully serve as an abstract ideal, a useful spur, remaining forever impossible to operationalise' (O'Connell and Radloff 1995: 59). So, should we abandon our attempts to care for the whole person, or should we continue to try to meet patients' diverse health care needs? Let us explore the relationship between holism and the psychological aspects of care in greater detail.

Holism and psychological care

In its simplest terms, psychological care is the part of holistic caring that responds to people's psychological needs. If holistic care is an ideal to be sought after, then in an attempt to translate what may be an abstract ideal into reality we must, amongst other activities, attempt to assess psychological needs accurately and deliver psychological care. It follows that if psychological care, as an element of holistic care, is not delivered, the patient on the receiving end could be described as not having been cared for. So what do we mean when we talk about 'psychological needs' and 'psychological care'?

Psychological needs

Psychological needs can be described as human needs relating to emotional, behavioural, and cognitive functioning. In other words, they are to do with feeling, doing, and thinking. In Chapter 1, we introduced Maslow's theory of human motivation, in which he viewed all human needs, apart from those ensuring physical survival, to be psychological in nature. For example, we need to feel safe, loved, and accepted, and intellectually stimulated. Hence, we all have psychological needs that, in an ideal world, are satisfied all of the time. Clearly, we do not live in such an ideal world. It is natural to experience negative emotions such as fear or sadness, and to experience self-doubts, particularly following negative life events such as bereavement or being made redundant from work. We might alter our behaviour in response, perhaps by withdrawing from family and friends for a while. For the most part, though, if we have adequate support from those around us, we will be able to work through these difficult experiences and emotions and overcome them. Indeed, it is generally acknowledged that social support is a critical factor in determining whether someone will develop and especially recover from a mental health problem (see, for example, NICE 2009). The same is true of psychological needs in illness, if they are identified and addressed by carers. In sum, those needs which relate to human emotional, behavioural and cognitive functioning may be referred to as psychological needs, and the process of intervening and attending to those needs may be referred to as psychological care. But what happens to our psychological needs when we are removed from our usual sources of support, such as when we are ill and admitted to hospital?

Psychological needs in illness

Psychological needs are particularly active and relevant when someone becomes ill and in need of health care services. One of the difficulties in understanding the concept of psychological need in illness is the range of terminology used, with terms such as 'psychological need', 'psychosocial need' and 'emotional need' used synonymously. As long ago as 1986, Fleming pointed out that nurses had difficulty in defining needs that are not physical, and highlighted the tendency of nurses to use vague terminology to cover any deficits in this area.

More recently, Priest (1999) asked student and qualified nurses for their views on the meaning of 'psychological needs' in nursing. Responses suggest that psychological needs are seen as primarily emotional (to do with feelings) and cognitive (to do with thoughts), although social needs were also deemed relevant. For example, one student commented that psychological needs are, 'looking after the [patient's] mind as well as the body, understand what they're thinking, what their emotions might be, and trying to put those right as well as the body'.

A possible definition of psychological need in an illness/health care/nursing context is, 'an expression of psychological functioning that characterises a personal longing, want, or wish, or, alternatively, an expression of distress, deprivation or inadequacy' (Bach 1995: 31). Psychological functioning, within this definition, might encompass social needs, and the need for independence, control, information, social interaction, privacy and dignity. Such needs might manifest themselves in a range of behavioural expressions that are unique to each individual, but it is possible to recognise misery, fear, anxiety, frustration, loss of motivation and loss of confidence. As a participant in Priest's study commented, we can sometimes identify psychological needs through behaviours:

> the words and what they're telling you, and their actions, if they don't want to get out of bed, or they don't seem to be taking any notice of what's going on around them, they don't want anything to eat, or drink or anything like that.

It is widely acknowledged that negative emotions, cognitions, and behaviours, can be activated in physical illness or following injury, especially where admission to hospital is required, and that these in turn can have a negative impact upon recovery. As long ago as 1976, Wilson-Barnett demonstrated that hospital patients frequently suffer psychological distress, and that this is often exacerbated by factors intrinsic to being in hospital, such as anticipating painful treatments or procedures, lack of information and being away from work and family. Nichols (2003) provides us with a comprehensive list of common psychological reactions to illness, based upon his extensive clinical observations. These are summarised in Figure 3.2.

> - Shock at the event and its implications.
> - Threat and anxiety.
> - Post-traumatic stress reactions.
> - Distress at being in hospital and with treatments.
> - Lowered personal control.
> - Damage to self image.
> - Loss of self worth.
> - Grief.
> - Anger.
> - Depression.
> - Denial.
> - Exaggerated independence or dependency.
> - Partner crisis, stress and guilt.

Figure 3.2 Common psychological reactions to illness and hospitalisation (Nichols 2003)

Reproduced and adapted from Nichols, K. (2003) *Psychological Care for Ill and Injured People,* p. 45, with kind permission of Open University Press/McGraw-Hill Education.

Nichols also provides us with detailed descriptions of these responses, illustrated with case study material, because although general patterns of psychological needs and responses in illness might be predicted, individuals will respond in unique ways when they become ill. According to Bor, Gill, Miller and Evans (2009: 41), such individual response is 'diverse, unique, and unpredictable in its nature and intensity'. As an experienced nurse in Priest's (2001) study commented:

> You can't uniformly say, well, every patient who comes in, we'll do this for, because they might react to it differently, so you're going back to the concept of holism . . . we might do this for one patient, but it might not work for others, we'll have to see how it goes.

Clearly, then, there is a relationship between illness and psychological need. This is a two-way relationship; not only may a person's psychological state affect the onset and outcome of physical illness, but illness may also create psychological problems that can impede recovery. Nichols (1993) argues more strongly that there is a causal relationship between illness and psychological need: 'Serious illness, disability or disfigurement *inevitably* cause psychological reactions or psychological disturbance' (Nichols 1993: 46).

Thus, broad reactions will be amplified when patients' conditions are serious or where the outcome is unlikely to be positive. For example, Low *et al.* (2007) identified that the most common reactions and concerns in advanced illness such as cancer are coping with uncertainty and unpredictability, lack of control and fear of dependency. Indeed, we might reasonably expect all patients admitted to hospital, regardless of the severity of their problem, to be anxious, and to need information about their problem, how it will be explored and how it will be treated. However, there will also be individual variations in the nature and degree of anxiety experienced by patients, and in the kinds of information they will need to reduce this anxiety.

Reflection point

What factors might influence patients' unique responses when they are admitted to hospital?

Patients' responses will depend on a number of factors such as those in Figure 3.3; some are personal factors, such as individual coping strategies, and some are external or situational factors, such as the amount of information provided by carers.

Do all patients have psychological needs?

If we agree with Nichols and indeed Maslow, then not only all patients, but also all people do indeed have psychological needs that must be satisfied if they are to achieve fulfilment in their everyday lives. Thus there are likely to be psychological consequences of all illness, no matter how trivial. It has been suggested, for example, that patients admitted for day surgery, by definition for relatively minor conditions, experience much anxiety but receive inadequate psychological support (Mitchell 2002, 2005; Bellani 2008). A key difficulty, according to Nichols (2003: 36), is that, particularly in the UK, we live in a 'culture of masked reactions', which encourages patients to hide their true feelings and to appear positive, even when faced with difficult diagnoses or uncertain prognoses. This tendency is illustrated by two nurses in Priest's study:

> Some people are very good at hiding it, some . . . people think they don't want to be a burden to anyone, or they don't want to bother anybody, they won't let out their emotions, what they're feeling, because it may bother somebody, put extra on the staff, so they keep it hidden away.

- Patients' previous experiences of illness and health care, their experience of being cared for and the outcome of this previous treatment and care.
- Patients' knowledge and beliefs about their illness, how it was caused, and how it should be treated.
- How patients sees themselves, and the degree of control they perceive they have over their illness.
- Patients' tolerance to stress and the range and efficacy of their coping strategies.
- The degree of social and emotional support available to the patients (this may be actual support, or the level of support perceived to be available by the patient).
- The way the individual is treated by health care staff.
- The physical care environment, which may contribute to sensory deprivation.
- The culture and beliefs of staff in the care environment and their working practices and priorities.

Figure 3.3 Factors affecting individual patients' response to illness

Reproduced and adapted from Priest, H., (2010). 'Effective psychological care for physically ill patients in hospital', Nursing Standard 24(44), 52, with kind permission of RCN Publishing Company.

So while we might expect our patients to have psychological needs that must be identified and addressed, we could infer that because they are smiling and not in obvious distress, then we do not need to take any particular action. This equates in some cases to 'psychological neglect' (Nichols 1993).

However, we must take care not to assume that experiencing a psychological need is always an undesirable state or deficiency that requires remedial action. A need is not necessarily a problem, provided it can be satisfied in an acceptable and timely manner, and may produce positive behaviours and emotions. Indeed, Maslow (1973: 379) described the fulfilment of psychological needs as enabling 'the fullest height to which the human being can attain'. Thus, a desire to address and rectify needs and to 'make the patient feel better' may in some cases be misplaced and misguided, and deny the patient the opportunity for personal growth and learning arising out of the illness experience.

Why caring for psychological needs is important

As we shall see, providing an effective response to patients' psychological needs is not only crucial for the patients themselves, but is also important to those providing that care. To care effectively, health care professionals need to be able to identify and respond appropriately to patients' unique expressions of psychological need; this process may be referred to as psychological care. Although there may not be a universal agreement about what psychological need and care actually means, we can draw on evidence about what happens when patients' psychological needs are not met. Unfortunately, despite much knowledge about the importance of good psychological caregiving, there has long existed evidence to suggest that health care professionals are not good at attending to psychologically based needs. Harrison (2001: 47), for example, pointed out that 'despite increasing recognition that psychological processes play a significant role in predisposing individuals to certain illnesses, and acknowledgment of their influence on morbidity and mortality rates', in practice the emotional and psychological aspects of a patient's care tend to be forgotten.

In confirmation, as part of its role, the Parliamentary and Health Service Ombudsman listens to, investigates and responds to concerns and complaints about the health service in England, and publishes an annual report (http://www.ombudsman.org.uk/about-us/publications/annual-reports). Many of the cases investigated focus on poor communication and information-sharing between professional and patient, and between professionals, rather than on poor clinical treatments or physical care. The nature and amount of information offered to patients and relatives frequently gives cause for concern, leaving them feeling anxious, frustrated, and angry.

Specific studies carried out over the past three decades provide further evidence. For example, Johnson (1982) found that although nurses and patients could agree on the general range of issues likely to be worrying patients, in practice nurses could not identify their patients' specific worries. Farrell (1991) similarly found little correspondence between patients' and their nurses' views of their individual needs. Mitchell (1997) agreed that nurses were poor at assessing the presence of anxiety in their patients. More recently, Harrison (2001) confirmed that clinicians frequently fail to recognise patients' emotional needs in clinical practice, and where they do recognise them, the majority feel unable to address them appropriately. Sometimes, this is because they are fearful of what they see as 'mental health problems' or because they do not want to create emotional distress in themselves, but more often it is to do with preferring to attend to concrete physical needs that they see as more amenable to intervention.

Other studies support such findings and make a clear link between physical illness and psychological problems. For example, Ramirez and House (1998) found that 12 per cent of people referred to medical outpatient clinics have a psychological basis for their problems, while around 25 per cent of patients in general hospitals have adjustment and mood disorders (Harrison 2001). Lane *et al.* (2002, cited in Nichols 2003: 82) found that symptoms of depression and anxiety are prevalent and persistent during the first year following a myocardial infarction, and Hemingway and Marmot (1999, cited in Nichols 2005: 27) found that the probability of a second heart attack increased with emotional disarray and lack of support. Physical health problems such as diabetes, cancer and cardiac conditions are frequently accompanied by psychological problems (Harrison 2001). The Centre for Economic Performance's Mental Health Policy Group known as the Layard Report (LSE, 2006) found that one third of clinical presentations in primary care are psychological, while clinical depression accounts for 12 per cent of total non fatal illness (Utsün *et al.* 2004, cited in Bor *et al.* 2009: 41). Some specific illnesses, such as Parkinson's disease and epilepsy, have psychological difficulties as part of their usual presentation (Harrison 2001), with depression, for example, being a central feature of multiple sclerosis.

The impact of failing to address such psychological needs when they occur alongside or as an integral part of a physical illness can be enormous. Priest's (2001, 2002) study showed that when patients do not receive appropriate psychological care, they experience uncertainty, are not in control, and feel anxious, as summarised by one participant:

> When my grand-dad was in hospital recently . . . it was a surgical ward, and the staff hardly spoke to us, there were people around and they don't tell you what they're doing, and you worry then because you don't know what's going on, and that's part of psychological care, isn't it?

More recently, Nichols (2005) described a survey in which less than 10 per cent of patients interviewed following cardiac surgery said anything positive when asked whether psychological care had been provided to them during their treatment and care. Reviewing studies conducted during the 1970s and 1980s, Nichols (1993, 2003) identified problems arising when patients' psychological needs were not adequately identified or met. These included:

- delayed or prolonged recovery from illness;
- increased mortality rates;
- reduced compliance with treatment or medical advice;
- increased use of medical and nursing services;
- the development of serious mental health problems.

Hence, as summarised by Bor *et al.* (2009: 43) 'To ignore the psychological care of the patient is no longer an option in the modern, accountable health care setting'. The work of Layard (LSE 2006), cited above, has been particularly helpful in enhancing our understanding of psychological difficulties. Layard showed that psychological problems such as depression and anxiety are more likely to cause unhappiness than physical ill health factors such as pain and immobility, and are as likely to cause as much unhappiness as poverty. Layard's influential work led to the 'Increasing Access to Psychological Therapies' (IAPT) strategy, aimed at reducing the personal and economic distress of psychological ill health through the timely provision of psychological support in the community. This strategy led to an increase in the number and type of trained psychological therapists. Clearly, then, if everyday psychological difficulties have such devastating effects, it is particularly important to identify and address them in anxiety-provoking situations such as illness or hospitalisation.

The positive effects of psychological care

In contrast, research suggests that when psychological needs are met, recovery is improved, use of medical services is reduced and patient satisfaction improves. Devine (1992), for example, reviewed 191 studies to explore the effectiveness of what she termed 'psycho-educational care'; these included studies where psychological support or education was provided to adult surgical patients. Devine concluded that appropriate interventions contributed to improved recovery, shorter hospital stay, reduced pain, and reduced psychological distress. Linden's (1996) meta-analysis of 23 studies showed that patients with coronary artery disease who received specific psychosocial treatment (such as education, counselling and relaxation therapy) showed greater reductions in psychological distress as well as heart rate, blood pressure and cholesterol level than those who did not. Additionally, those who did not receive psychosocial treatment had greater mortality rates and more recurrence of cardiac problems. More recently, Di Blasi *et al.* (2001) also conducted a systematic review of the literature to explore whether the quality of the doctor–patient relationship had any impact on treatment outcomes, independent of the treatment itself. Their review suggested that doctors who provide support, reassurance and positive information (and are thus more humane and compassionate in their approach) are more effective in enhancing health outcomes than those who adopt a more formal and factual style. In Priest's (2001) study, nurses felt that when patients received timely and effective psychological care, their well-being was maintained or improved and anxiety reduced; they experienced a feeling of safety and were empowered within the constraints of their illness.

Providing effective attention to psychological needs is also important for the carer providing that attention. When effective and timely psychological care has been delivered, it is experienced by the nurse as a pleasurable moment, in which a connection with the experience of the patient is felt, and one that brings personal reward, as illustrated by a junior nurse in Priest's study:

> During the experience I felt a sense of doing something worthwhile and useful to the patient in a way that doing something like bandaging a leg or applying a dressing is seen as necessary to the patient's recovery. Little things [are] not really a necessity to the patient but in terms of personal pleasure it is worth a whole lot more.

In contrast, when psychological care is not delivered, whether due to external or internal reasons, the experience is of guilt and frustration, as shown by other nurses in the same study: 'You're not caring, you're just providing, that's the best way of putting it'. In some cases this frustration turns to a sense of failure in the job and the experience of personal distress:

> I think that's what causes me a lot of psychological distress really, the fact that I don't feel that I'm providing the best care that I can, to people that are passing through our ward . . . When I can't carry that through I think that's when I get really, really dissatisfied with the job.

The consequences of giving and receiving psychological care are considered further in Chapter 4.

When does a psychological need become a psychological problem, and how do we tell the difference?

Nichols (1993, 2003) has spoken of 'neglect' and 'psychological damage' occurring in hospitals caused by staff who have not attended appropriately to the psychological needs of their physically ill patients. In some cases, lack of attention to patients' psychological needs can lead to them developing more serious psychological or mental health problems.

To be mentally healthy, we need to experience a balance between all aspects of our life (including social, physical, spiritual, and emotional elements), feel positive about ourselves and others, meet the demands of everyday life, and make appropriate life choices. If we have a psychological or mental health problem (sometimes described as a mental disorder, psychiatric illness, or mental illness), our daily life and/or that of others is likely to be adversely affected to some degree. According to the American Psychiatric Association (2000), a mental health problem, or mental disorder, is 'a clinically significant behavioural or psychological syndrome or pattern . . . that is associated with present distress or disability or with a significantly increased risk of suffering, death, pain, disability, or an important loss of freedom . . .'. Put more simply, a mental health problem exists when there is a change in an individual's emotions, behaviour and thinking to the extent that day-to-day life, activities and relationships are adversely affected.

Mental health problems are extremely common. It is estimated that at least a quarter of the population will experience a mental health problem at some point in their lives, with costly consequences – mental health problems represent up to 23 per cent of the health care costs in the UK – and they are the largest single cause of illness (NICE 2011).

What causes mental health problems?

We can think of mental health and mental illness as extreme ends of a continuum. Where an individual is at any one time on that continuum is determined by a range of factors such as:

- predisposing biological or genetic factors;
- factors that increase a person's vulnerability to stress, such as adverse childhood experiences, poor coping strategies, or lack of support;
- external stressful events or 'triggers'.

Often, a person can cope perfectly well with a huge number of difficulties, but may reach the point where a new difficulty, even if minor, becomes 'the straw that breaks the camel's back'. Some mental health problems, however, are likely to develop regardless of a person's day-to-day experience. These include degenerative organic disorders such as dementia, where changes in the brain associated with ageing cause irreversible deterioration in cognitive functioning and eventually changes in behaviour and personality. Other common mental health problems include mood disorders (such as depression); anxiety disorders (such as generalised anxiety, phobias, and obsessive-compulsive disorders); and psychoses (major and severe conditions such as schizophrenia and bipolar disorder).

No-one is born with a mental health problem, although it is thought that people may inherit a genetic predisposition to develop certain conditions, such as schizophrenia. In many cases, mental health problems will resolve themselves with or without intervention from health care professionals. In some cases, however, intervention is required; this might take the form of a 'talking therapy' such as counselling or psychotherapy; a physical therapy, such as antidepressant medication, or a therapy focusing on people's thought processes and behaviour, such as cognitive behaviour therapy (CBT). With more serious mental health problems such as schizophrenia, it is likely that long-term intervention, combining medication and other psychological and social interventions will be needed, and there is likely to be a progressive downhill course over time.

Clearly, when someone requires this level of intervention, it is beyond the scope of non-specialists to offer it, but recognising that someone has developed or is at risk of developing a mental health problem and knowing where and how to refer that patient for specialist help is vital. Making this distinction between a psychological need activated by illness, and a more serious mental health problem, forms part of a comprehensive assessment process, which will be explored further in Chapter 6.

Referring on: The Role of Specialist Practitioners

In Chapter 4, we shall see that effective psychological care can be delivered at many levels and by practitioners with various levels of experience and expertise. Crucially, however, every health care practitioner must have the self knowledge and self awareness to recognise their limitations; to recognise when an aspect of care delivery has exceeded their current level of skill or knowledge, and to know what action should be taken to secure an appropriate referral.

There are a number of specialist practitioners whose expertise may be required by hospital patients. These include advocates, counsellors, liaison mental health nurses, health psychologists, clinical psychologists and psychiatrists. We now review the roles of these specialists, both in furthering our understanding of psychological needs and care and in selecting appropriate referral options.

Advocate

Advocates represent, support and encourage people who are in any way disadvantaged or vulnerable to ensure that their basic rights are met. This may include people with intellectual disabilities or those who may lack mental capacity due to a head injury, a neurological condition, or a serious mental health problem such as dementia. In this way, they empower people to meet their own needs, with appropriate support. The Mental Capacity Act (2005) requires an Independent Advocate Service to be in place for adults who lack mental capacity and have no appropriate friends or family to consult in situations where providing or withholding serious medical treatment is at issue. Clearly, advocates could have an important role to play in ensuring that the psychological needs of vulnerable and unsupported people are met.

Counsellor

The NHS employs a range of staff who provide counselling to patients, sometimes working with specific groups such as people with cancer or genetic disorders, but sometimes working more generically. We explore basic counselling skills further in Chapter 6, but the primary role of a professional counsellor is actively listening to patients' difficulties or distress, seeing their difficulties from the patient's point of view, and helping them to see things more clearly. It rarely, if ever, involves giving advice (NHS Careers, http://www.nhscareers. nhs.uk/atoz.shtml). Many counsellors in the UK are accredited by and registered with the

British Association of Counsellors and Psychotherapists (BACP, http://www.bacp.co.uk/information/education/whatiscounselling.php).

Liaison mental health nurse

A liaison mental health nurse is a qualified mental health nurse who works to bridge the divide between physical health and mental health care settings. Liaison nurses often work in settings such as accident and emergency departments, where they might, for example, take referrals to see people who have self-harmed or attempted suicide. They also work in oncology and obstetrics and gynaecology settings, and also with people with HIV Aids, in cardiac rehabilitation, and with people with conditions such as chronic fatigue syndrome, body image disturbance, and post-traumatic stress disorder (Regel and Roberts 2002).

Health psychologist

Health psychologists use psychological principles to promote changes in people's attitudes, behaviour and thinking about health and illness. They are normally educated to Masters or Doctoral level and can help, for example, when people wish to give up smoking, improve their diet, or reduce alcohol intake, but they can also help people prepare for stressful or painful procedures, and cope with the psychological effects of illness (BPS 2010).

Clinical psychologist

Clinical psychologists also use psychological theory to assess and intervene when patients have psychological and mental health problems such as anxiety or depression, or more serious mental illnesses such as schizophrenia or dementia. They are normally educated to Doctoral level. There is some overlap here with the role of psychiatrist (see below), although psychiatrists operate from a medical framework rather than a psychological perspective. A specific element of clinical psychologists' work is the psychological *formulation,* made following assessment and before intervention, during which a provisional psychological explanation is made of the patient's situation (Johnstone and Dallos 2006). Clinical psychologists also work with people with intellectual disabilities, eating disorders, and those experiencing relationship difficulties (BPS 2010).

Psychiatrist

Psychiatrists are medically trained doctors who have undergone further specialist training to deal with all aspects of people's mental health, although they will often specialise in areas such as adult mental health; intellectual disabilities; child and adolescent psychiatry; old age psychiatry; forensic psychiatry; or psychotherapy. They carry out detailed assessments of psychological functioning and can offer a range of interventions including different forms of psychotherapy and medication.

It must be noted that there may be conflicts in the way in which different professional groups construe the meaning of psychological care. At a recent psychology conference, for example, a clinical psychologist publicly questioned the rights of nurses to utilise psychological skills which were deemed to be the province of psychologists alone. Such misunderstandings about the nature of the work of the professional groups contributing to the care of physically ill patients can do little to enhance the quality of the care that they receive. Good inter-professional communication is needed to minimise the potential impact of such professional differences on care delivery.

Summary

In conclusion, we have seen that anyone experiencing an illness or disability that requires health care intervention, no matter how minor, requires psychological care. We have also seen that psychological needs that are not identified or unmet can lead to negative and serious consequences. We have noted that patients' responses to illness are unique and related to a number of internal (personal) and external (environmental) factors. It follows, then, that effective psychological care will be delivered when patients' unique psychological needs are met. In order to ensure that this happens, health care professionals must be skilled at assessing and monitoring patients' psychological state, and referring on to a specialist practitioner when required.

But how do we go about addressing psychological needs and delivering effective psychological care? In Chapter 4 we present a model for psychological caregiving, and in subsequent chapters we consider the personal qualities, skills and knowledge that underpin such care.

4   A model for psychological care

He who would do good to another must do it in minute particulars.

(William Blake 2001)

Introduction

In Chapter 3, we concluded that all people experiencing an illness or disability that requires health care intervention, no matter how minor, require psychological care. We saw that psychological needs, unless appropriately identified and met, can lead to undesirable and, in some cases, serious consequences for patients and carers alike. Hence the need for nurses and other health care staff to be skilled at identifying and responding to the psychological needs of their patients. So how can we understand what it is to provide effective psychological care?

This chapter will develop the discussion around the nature and dimensions of psychological need and psychological care introduced in Chapter 3. It will review some early research work carried out to define and explain the nature of psychological care. It will then draw on Nichols' (1993, 2003) seminal work and psychological care schemes and also on later research by Priest (1999a, 1999b, 2001, 2002a, 2002b, 2006, 2010) to discuss the prerequisites for effective psychological care delivery; the main components of psychological care; and the consequences of giving and receiving psychological care for both carers and patients.

Defining psychological care

As with attempts to define care, caring, holistic care, and psychological need, there is a lack of clarity and consensus in the definition of psychological care. Early definitions include those of Hyland and Donaldson (1989) and Wilson-Barnett (1988). Hyland and Donaldson suggested that psychological care involves looking after patients' psychological needs through a range of skills such as listening, observing, empathising and communicating, with the ultimate goal of alleviating psychological suffering. It could be argued, however, that these skills are fundamental to care generally and not specific to the delivery of psychological care. Wilson-Barnett (1988) felt that the psychological interventions typically used with physically ill people were information giving, teaching, and counselling, and that carers must be able to assess and monitor patients' psychological state so that they are able to identify problems and decide upon the appropriate intervention. This might include deciding that referral to other agencies is required. Rimon's (1979) early work, from a psychologist's perspective, provided more specificity and suggested that a nurse's psychological role was to anticipate and meet emotional needs, to establish a relationship, to communicate, and to encourage self-reliance and independence. Specific interventions identified as part of this psychological role included explaining hospital routines, policies and treatment regimes; recognising the need for psychological or psychiatric help and making the appropriate referral; demonstrating acceptance and willingness to listen; and calming, comforting, advising, counselling and giving hope. Thus, as long ago as the 1970s, Rimon's guidance made clear that effective psychological care drew upon both the personal qualities and interpersonal skills of the carer. We explore these elements further in Chapters 5 and 6.

Nichols (1985), also from a clinical psychology standpoint, suggested that psychological care 'involves giving direct assistance and continuing support to clients as they deal with the reactions to serious illness or injury' (Nichols 1985: 233), and should be a routine provision, not an added extra or a luxury provided only when time is available. However, giving direct assistance and support would seem to be integral components of a caring role, not luxury activities, highlighting once more the difficulty of differentiating between general aspects of good care and psychological care.

We can see from these early attempts to define psychological care that there is some consensus about its key components, namely assessment, information giving, listening, and responding to emotions. Nichols' (1993) original scheme of psychological care (Figure 4.1) provides a useful starting point for exploring these dimensions more fully.

Nichols (1985, 1993, 2003) is one of few writers to have developed a formal scheme or model of psychological care in physical illness, which serves both as a guide to the delivery of psychological care in practice and to the teaching and learning of psychological caregiving skills. In 1993, based on his extensive research and observations as a clinical psychologist within a renal care setting, Nichols identified the central elements of psychological care as: informational or educational care; emotional care; basic counselling; and advocacy, as shown in Figure 4.1. However, in addition, Nichols stressed that assessment and monitoring of a patients' psychological state was a prerequisite for effective psychological care and that staff must know how and when to refer a patient for more specialist psychological support. Finally, Nichols' scheme acknowledged that psychological caregiving could be demanding and stressful and that staff should have the opportunity to participate in staff support systems.

Developing this research and observations further, Nichols (2003) moved on to categorise the elements of psychological care into three levels, according to who might carry them out and the level of knowledge and skill required. The three levels and the components within them are outlined in Figure 4.2.

- Monitoring patients' psychological state
  - (this may lead to referral for more specialist psychological therapy)
- Psychological care:
  - informational/educational care
  - emotional care
  - basic counselling
  - advocacy
- Staff self-care

Figure 4.1 Elements of Nichols' (1993) psychological care scheme

Adapted from Nichols, K. A. (1993) *Psychological Care in Physical Illness* (2nd edn), (p. 51). London: Chapman and Hall.

> **Level 1 Awareness**
> * awareness of psychological issues
> * patient-centred listening
> * patient-centred communication
> * awareness of patients' psychological state; relevant action
>
> **Level 2 Intervention**
> * monitoring and recording psychological state
> * information and education
> * emotional care
> * counselling
> * support/advocacy/referral
>
> **Level 3**
> * psychological therapy
> ....
>
> **Self care**

Figure 4.2 The components of psychological care (Nichols 2003)

Reproduced from Nichols, K. (2003) *Psychological Care for Ill and Injured People* (p. 6). With kind permission of Open University Press/McGraw-Hill Education.

As with Nichols' earlier psychological care scheme, we can see here that self care in the provision of psychological care is an important element and that assessment and monitoring remain important components at Levels 1 and 2.

Reflection point

Drawing on the levels of psychological care in Figure 4.2, in which, if any, of these three levels of psychological care would you expect the following staff to be skilled, and why? (You may like to refer back to Chapter 3 for descriptions of some of these roles).

* A first-year student nurse working in a medical ward.
* A psychological therapist.
* A senior physiotherapist.
* A junior doctor.
* A newly qualified children's nurse.
* A clinical psychologist.
* A mental health liaison nurse.

In summary, Level 1 represents having an awareness of the patient's psychological needs, and arguably all health care providers must operate as a minimum at this level (Hoyt 1995). Nichols (2003) felt that 'awareness' was something that should be achievable by all staff, no matter how junior or inexperienced, and arguably, even in training, health care students should receive adequate input on observation, listening and communication skills so that they can be aware of a patient's psychological needs and inform a more senior member of staff if they experience concerns.

Level 2 represents a more active level of intervention, but includes activities of relevance to all health care staff, such as providing support, giving information, providing health education, and referring on to other agencies as required. However, it may be that some skills listed under Level 2, such as counselling, only develop with experience and after attending appropriate training programmes, and are more relevant therefore to staff such as an experienced nurse, a mental health liaison nurse, a psychological therapist, or a member of medical staff.

Finally, Level 3 represents an advanced level of psychological support in the form of psychological therapy, likely to be carried out only by very specialist staff such as psychological therapists, clinical psychologists or psychiatrists within most hospital and primary care settings. We explore some of the contexts in which this level of therapy might be used in Chapter 8.

It is important to note that the word 'therapy', originating from the Greek *therapeia,* means 'a service', and is generally taken to mean a service to the sick. Thus to be 'therapeutic' implies doing something that is beneficial, restorative or curative and leads to a positive or healing outcome. Therefore, although specific 'psychological therapy' will be beyond the remit of the everyday carer, some of the knowledge and skills used by such specialists can be drawn upon to inform the repertoire of everyday practitioners, and thus all practitioners can be therapeutic. Essentially, according to Nichols (2005), psychological care differs from psychological therapy in that it is primarily a *preventive* activity. Try the exercise below to identify your own therapeutic role.

Action point

Reflect on recent practice experience and identify a carer–patient intervention (in which you were the carer) that was, in your view, therapeutic.

Describe the intervention.

What did you hope to achieve?

Describe the outcome.

Identify the specific elements of the intervention that made it 'therapeutic'.

Was any part of the intervention preventive?

The nurse theorist Hildegarde Peplau (1952) referred to nursing as a therapeutic process, and Ersser (1990) studied the therapeutic effect of nursing. He concluded that nurses' appearance, attitudes and manner can be therapeutic as they have an impact on patients' well-being. Furthermore, when nurses genuinely express emotions, make themselves available, and convey confidence, patients experience these elements as at least as important as specific nursing procedures. It may be that you identified such actions and attributes within your reflections.

Returning to Nichols' (2003) components of psychological care, it is important to note that psychological care delivery cannot be delivered effectively unless staff themselves are cared for, and know when to refer patients for more specialist help. Finally, within Nichols' model, all staff need to be sufficiently self-aware to know the limits of their ability, and to know how and to whom to refer. We explore self- awareness and self care further in Chapter 5.

In the continuing search for clarity regarding the meaning of 'psychological care', Priest (1999a, 1999b, 2001, 2002, 2006) conducted research attempting to describe and define psychological care as it operates within nursing. This research included an exercise in which nurses completed the sentence: 'To me, psychological care in nursing means . . .'.

Action point

Before reading the results of the above survey, try the exercise yourself, in relation to your own health care profession.

Complete the sentence 'to me, psychological care means . . .'.

In Priest's study, a total of 91 descriptions were produced, which were organised into 18 descriptive categories by a content analysis process informed by Denscombe (1998) and Burnard (1994a, 1994b). The 18 categories are listed in Table 4.1., with the frequency given for each item by number of participants. Did your suggestions match up?

From this analysis, the aspect upon which there is most agreement is that psychological care is related to understanding and responding to aspects of patients' psychological functioning. Related to this belief is the notion that psychological care makes an important contribution to holistic care, as discussed in Chapter 3. As mentioned by some of the respon-

Table 4.1 Descriptive categories derived from sentence completion exercise

Category	Number of items
Psychological functioning	21
Holistic	16
Listening/counselling/facilitating emotional expression	10
Complementary to physical care	10
An integral part of physical care	6
Empathy	5
Information and its effects	5
Spiritual aspects	5
Well-being	4
Sexual/body image	4
Coming to terms	3
Individuality	3
Referral	2
Social aspects	2
Nurse's role	2
Assessing (and planning)	2
Love	1
Time	1

dents, it involves: 'Caring for the effects that illness has on the mind' and 'Ensuring that the patient's psychological well-being is given as much attention as their physical needs'.

In some cases, psychological care is thought to subsume what might be considered separate elements of holistic care, such as spiritual, sexual and social care: 'Maintaining emotional, social, spiritual, and sexual well-being to complement physical care in order for the individual to achieve optimum health'.

The aim of psychological caregiving is less clear from this exercise, but may be directed towards the achievement of well-being, or, perhaps where well-being is not achievable, to a state of acceptance of changes brought about by physical illness such that: 'The person experiences a sense of well being relative to themselves' or is helped to 'come to terms with what is going to happen or has happened already'.

These nurses felt that psychological care was dependent upon role function more than on the performance of specific interpersonal skills or the presence of particular personal qualities. This being the case, it should be possible to equip every nurse with the ability to deliver essential psychological care, provided that it is viewed as part of the everyday nursing role.

The research also included interviews with qualified ('expert') and student ('novice') nurses (drawing on Benner's [1984] seminal work and analysed using Colaizzi's [1978] phenomenological approach to qualitative data analysis) to discover whether, in line with Nichols' proposals, different elements of psychological care were related to different levels of qualification and experience. Specifically, student nurses in training were compared with experienced nurses (qualified and practising for at least three years). Key findings are illustrated in Table 4.2.

In fact, as shown in Table 4.2, there was a high degree of agreement between what novices and experts thought psychological care involved, particularly around relationship building, emotional care, using the care environment, and advocacy, some of which were also evident in Nichols' (1993) original scheme. Interestingly, students identified more elements of psychological care than experienced nurses, perhaps suggesting that experienced nurses have

Table 4.2 Novice and expert nurses' perceptions of the meaning of psychological care

Novice	*Expert*
Using personal qualities	Self-awareness
Being available	'Being with' the patient
Comfort, safety, reassurance	
Advocacy	Advocacy
Relationship building	Relationship building
Counselling	Communication skills
Emotional care	Emotional care
Atmosphere in the care environment	Using the care environment
'Leaving the door open'	'Leaving the door open'
Picking up cues	
Involving relatives	
Timing/prioritising	
Distracting	
Constraints	Constraints
Information giving	

Reproduced and adapted from Novice and expert perceptions of psychological care and the development of psychological caregiving abilities, *Nurse Education Today* 19(7), Helena M. Priest, 1999. With permission from Elsevier.

internalised some of their psychological care activities in line with Benner's (1984) theory of nursing expertise. However, it was only the experienced nurses who highlighted the importance of information-giving as a discrete element of psychological care.

In sum, Priest's (2001) research confirmed Nichols' central concepts of assessment, information/education, emotional care, and counselling. An extended phenomenological description of psychological care was produced (Priest 2002) based on literature reviews, the sentence completion exercises described above, analysis of nursing curriculum content, reflective writing, and longitudinal interviews conducted over a two-year period. This description included the essential nature and experience of psychological needs, the nature of psychological caregiving, the pre-conditions for psychological caregiving, the consequences for the patient, and the experience of the nurse in giving and not giving psychological care. These findings are presented in the model shown in Figure 4.3.

We move on now to consider some of the preconditions of psychological caregiving, as identified in both Nichols' psychological care schemes (Figures 4.1. and 4.2) and in Priest's model of psychological care (Figure 4.3).

Pre-requisites for psychological care

Although the specific skills of assessment, information/educational care, and emotional care are fundamental to psychological care, it is equally important that a set of preconditions is in place, upon which the delivery of effective psychological care is contingent. The idea that effective psychological caregiving is contingent upon certain pre-conditions is not a novel one. Previous studies of caring have foreshadowed this idea in a range of ways. As early as 1979 Watson claimed her ten carative factors were preconditions for caring. Fisher and Tronto (1990) specifically identified the preconditions of time, material resources, knowledge and skill that influence the degree, quality, and extent of caring. Sadler (1997), too, identified as antecedents of caring competence, resources, intentional moral commitment, and experiential learning arising out of formal education and life experiences.

Nichols (2003) made clear that in order for the psychological care of all patients to be guaranteed within a hospital setting, certain factors needed to be in place. These include those listed in Figure 4.4.

Priest's research, too, identified a number of pre-requisites for effective psychological care delivery, as listed in Figure 4.5.

These two lists have many elements in common, and we will focus particularly on the following in the next section:

- a supportive clinical culture/environment;
- using role models;
- making time and space;
- addressing competing priorities.

These elements are illustrated with quotations from experienced and student nurses from a range of contexts in Priest's (2001) study. We also discuss the notion that effective psychological care can often be delivered through 'small acts', in accordance with the chapter opening quotation from the poet and artist William Blake. Further preconditions such as relationship building, intuition, reflection, and self awareness are discussed in more detail in Chapter 5.

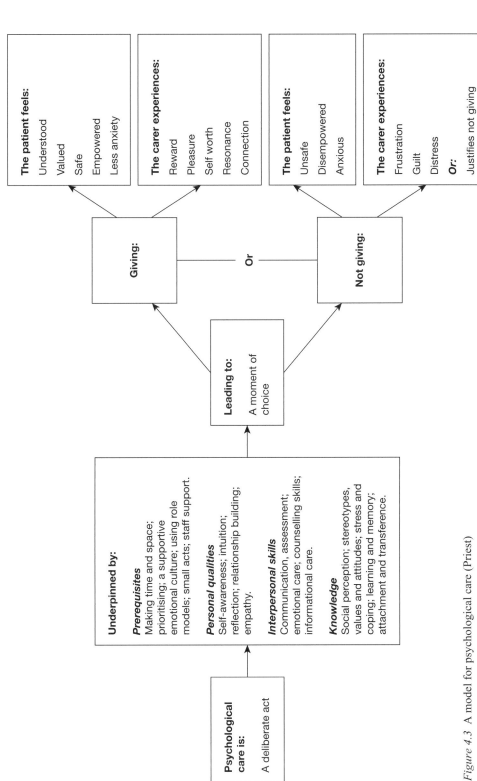

Figure 4.3 A model for psychological care (Priest)

- Training
- Explicit directions
- Allocation of 'psychological care duties'
- Materials
- Records of assessments/interventions
- Support from medical staff
- Referral systems in place
- Staff support

Figure 4.4 Pre-requisites for psychological care (Nichols 2003)

- Addressing competing priorities
- Making room for psychological care
- A supportive clinical culture
- Exposure to positive role models
- Pre-existing personal qualities
- Intuition
- Reflection
- The existence of at least a rudimentary nurse–patient relationship
- Care delivered through 'small acts'
- Ability to design and implement psychological care plans
- Being self-aware in relation to the possibility for care and the moment of choice

Figure 4.5 Pre-requisites for psychological care (Priest 2001, 2002)

A supportive clinical culture

It has long been recognised that ward contexts, hierarchies, power relations and ethos influence nurse–patient interactions (Jarrett and Payne 1995). It appears that no matter how willing individual practitioners might be, effective psychological care delivery is contingent on a care environment that is supportive of a strong focus on psychological needs. In areas where psychological care is viewed as less of a priority and a less legitimate type of work than carrying out physical tasks, nurses may be found wanting, and be criticised, if they have chosen to spend time with patients rather than completing practical activities (Muxlow 1995). Even in areas where sympathy with psychological caring might be expected, such conflicts exist. In James's (1992) study of hospice care, for example, nurses would, after spending time sitting talking to patients, declare that they must 'go and do some work now', indicating the need to perform physical tasks. The emotional component of caring had an ambivalent status, in part because it was invisible. The culture similarly influences the extent to which staff support and care are viewed as desirable or necessary, and hence determines the provision, or otherwise, of a framework for such support. These ideas are confirmed in a study by Rytterström *et al.* (2009) where nurses described hospital wards that have a caring culture as being 'homelike'. Furthermore, those people who are or appear to be 'in charge' or are 'strong personalities' transmit the dominant culture and socialise the staff into philosophies that are supportive, or otherwise, of psychological caregiving, as illustrated in Priest's (2006) study: 'It's leadership isn't it, that says whether there's good psychological care or not'.

Sadly, it appears that such a culture is not always in place, although sometimes this is due to the nature and pace of the work rather than unwillingness. For example, student nurses in Priest's study commented:

> It's how the ward approaches it, I mean the surgical ward's main priority was get somebody from theatre, make sure their obs [observation of vital signs] and everything are alright, get them home for the next one to go in.

> It [psychological care] wouldn't be the first thing, no. Keeping the place running ship shape, everyone seen to, bed bathed, dressed, fed, toileted, all those things. Observations and tests and what have you, because that's what the doctor would demand, when he comes round . . .

Sometimes, individuals are able to challenge the culture if it seems unsupportive of psychological caregiving, but this can carry some risks of being alienated by other staff members, and in the case of students, of receiving negative appraisals that might affect their future progress, as illustrated below:

> There was one gentleman sitting out of bed, an amputee, and he didn't want to sit out of bed, he'd been out for hours and he was feeling cold, and there was a slipper off his foot . . . so he was a bit miserable, but I went and reported it to the nurse that he wanted to get back into bed and she said he has to stay out because of his lungs. . . . So I went back and told him that she wouldn't let [him] . . . and he wasn't very happy, said that she was very hard, and I said well I'll get you a dressing gown and put your slipper on, that's all I can do . . . [I wondered] whether I should have taken his temperature, but I would have made myself an enemy on the ward probably [laughs]. It's only because she didn't have the full picture, I had a bit more [information] about him being cold. She just thought he had to sit out, he was just playing up.

Students are in a vulnerable position as their progress and performance is constantly monitored and evaluated by their experienced colleagues. There can be conflict between providing care and risking 'making enemies' of the people who have the power to determine their progress on their course. Rytterström *et al.* (2009) confirmed that nurses sometimes had to struggle to adapt to a ward's culture in order to be accepted, and to identify allies within the environment who see things in the same way as they do. Not every clinical environment considers psychological caregiving as high priority, and to deliver psychological care in such an environment requires a questioning and assertive stance. The prevailing culture is powerful, and individuals have to work hard to maintain and defend their own beliefs and priorities when they find themselves in a conflicting and dominant emotional culture. While recognising that challenging the established culture is potentially risky, nurses in Priest's study nevertheless saw this as an activity that is sometimes necessary to enhance psychological care. Failure to challenge might result in them absorbing and accepting without question policies and practices that they perceive as being unsupportive of psychological care.

The presence of positive role models

Linked to the nature of the care environment, experienced staff act as role models for junior staff and students, and provide a means for observing and considering the appropriateness of particular behaviours (Priest 2006). Much of nursing knowledge, for example, is invisible, but it can be learned by watching other more experienced nurses at work (Biley 2005). Henderson (2002) pointed out that student and junior nurses learn their role through professional socialisation, in which they become immersed in the norms and expectations of the culture they are in. Observing professional reference groups enables them to gain clarity about their own social identity and emerging role. In Priest's (2001, 2006) study, nurses only considered role models to be those nurses to whom they were exposed in clinical practice, and to a lesser extent, the patients they cared for; they did not identify nurse educators as contributing to the development of these abilities or facilitating the learning of caring, whether these teachers were encountered in academic settings or in clinical areas. Students in particular emphasised the importance of role models as an expected and actual source of becoming an effective psychological caregiver:

> You learn things from people, how to talk to . . . people . . . you think well maybe I'll try that. See what they do and try it for yourself.

> You gain off other people . . . that's what I've found in the first few months of being here, it's the other people, you take on their approach . . . and you think, well, I could have done it that way, but I didn't think about it.

Role modelling is a two-way process, and experienced staff need to recognise their own influence as role models, as experienced nurses commented:

> I think a lot of it you hope passes on to that person just by example, by the way you deal with people and treat people, you know it's . . . hard to teach people that . . . I think that is very difficult, actually, trying to teach people.

> I think though, the only way they can learn from us is by example, plus we do talk to them a lot about how we cope with different situations . . . and hopefully that's how they learn . . . We just tell them what we did in that situation, and I'm always very wary, I say to them that everybody . . . works in a different way, and that's the way it should be.

Role models provide the means for making distinctions between good and poor care. In order to learn from them, it is necessary to be able to discriminate between good and poor ones:

> If you see a nurse who's doing something which you think is awful then you tend to remember that more than a good nurse.

> If you watch some nurses, and know how abrupt they are with the patient, you think, I don't want to be like that ever, I think as a student nurse as well you see that. You see the bad role models and you see the ones that are good, [and find] your own way of doing that. And it's hard to define because . . . it comes from something that's within.

> I can identify a good model and a bad one, fortunately, so I'm hoping I won't fall into bad habits.

> I think you just observe, and you pick bits . . . and this is what I'm going to be like when I get there, you know, when I'm qualified . . . I'll have a bit of her, and a bit of her, and a bit of her.

Making time and space

Although effective psychological care is often delivered as a by-product of physical care activities, it does not always happen automatically; sometimes space and time have to be created specifically for it. Both 'timeliness' of interventions and the need to 'make room' for care have previously been identified in the literature. Chipman (1991), for example, specifically identified meeting patients' needs in a timely fashion as an important prerequisite for caring, and indeed the patients in Kent *et al.*'s (1996) study of unmet psychological needs identified the need for more staff time. However, what was apparent in this study was that the issue was not to do with lack of time but more to do with identifying and responding to needs at the appropriate time, the time when it was needed and acceptable to the patient. Furthermore, there was a sense that in even the most highly pressurised of clinical environments, room could be made for psychological care, providing that there was a will on the part of the nurse to do so. As one nurse in Priest's (2001) study reflected:

> I think it's just giving them the time to express any problems they've got . . . it's the fact that we always make time to go into the quiet room to admit our patients, so if someone doesn't get a break because there's no-one on the ward then that's what happens.

Arguably, though, not taking a break is not an example of good self care, creating a dilemma for care staff. Hawkins and Hollinworth (2004) attempted to enhance the significance of making specific time for psychological care by leading workshops in which participating nurses were instructed to separate nursing tasks from time spent talking to patients. They were asked to create a set time to offer 'careful, sensitive listening, exploration of significant personal problems, and encouragement to recognize and express painful or disturbing thoughts and feelings' (p. 544). The content of the workshops focused on psychological theory and counselling skills (see Chapter 6). One year on following the workshops, some participants showed 'a major shift in understanding and provision of psychological support'. They reported that being able to offer psychological support had affected both how they felt and how they approached their patients, and in particular that they were more aware of patients' non-verbal cues that might indicate specific psychological needs. However, while the profile of psychological caregiving had been raised for all participants who had attended the workshop, some participants had been unwilling to implement the activities and had thus not changed their day-to- day practice. For some, this was a conscious decision (although the reasons remain largely unknown) and not necessarily because they had not recognised the potential benefits. Harrison (2001) too believed that protected time was central to psychological care interventions.

Sometimes, however, it is not simply a question of having the time or making the time, but of being able to seize the moment when psychological care is required and will be received, and delivering care at the patient's pace. It is therefore, linked to accurate identification of need:

> I feel that psychological needs should be met when and as required and not at a later date when the original need may have been ignored or forgotten.

> I've seen the staff nurse . . . she allows the person to express his fears and anxieties even down to the little bits, where's my dentures going to be when I come back [from the

operating theatre]. And she allows for that, she doesn't rush him, before she goes on to the next thing.

Conversely, there is a need to recognise when the time is not right for psychological caregiving: 'With her it was definitely, we'll stop now, I'll come back later and see if you want anything else, but at the moment we'll leave it as it is because you don't want to know'. The opportunistic nature of psychological care delivery is recognised; opportunities are taken to attend to psychological needs through the medium of physical care activities or routine procedures:

> I was able to establish a rapport with him just by following the admissions procedure.

> As I was taking a BP [blood pressure] I engaged in conversation with the patient. The more she told me about her life and illness the better I understood the far-reaching consequences of [the disease].

> Yes, just talking to a patient, sitting down for ten minutes . . . having a chat to them, you can get a lot of information from somebody. Yes, maybe if you're doing their obs [monitoring vital signs] you can have a chat to them.

However, when there is no obvious need for physical care, then it can be difficult to justify the provision of psychological care in its own right: 'Because no physical nursing care was needed, it became difficult to engage in conversation, apart from 'hello' and asking if she was alright'. Thus, opportunities for legitimately providing psychological care alongside physical care are welcomed:

> That's why I used to enjoy giving baths to patients . . . because that's the time when you've got ten or fifteen minutes with one patient one-to-one, and I really do feel that that is needed every day.

In sum, while psychological care is recognised as essential to well-being and recovery, it is not something that happens automatically, and carers need to capitalise on all opportunities to provide it, both alongside and in addition to physical care activities. Often this places demands on carers to juggle competing priorities in order to ensure that psychological needs are identified and met, as we outline in the next section.

Addressing competing priorities: the moment of choice

Deliberate caring does not just happen; it requires intentional action (Sadler 1997). Such action is predicated upon a moment of choice: 'Saying 'yes', attending to what is in front of us, is our decision to care. Saying 'no', not attending, separating ourselves, is deciding not to care' (Moccia 1990: 207). The concept of a moment of choice bears similarities to Watson's (1999) notion of the caring moment, in which the nurse creates an open space in which connectedness with the patient can occur. However, just as that connectedness can occur, so too can the open space, or opportunity, be rejected or ignored. As Brown *et al.* (1992: 34) suggested: 'Each one of us is free to reject the impulse to care, to reduce inter-actions to the level of abstract problem solving, to fence off our emotional response to the cared-for, and to assume the objective attitude'. The space that Watson (1999) has described can be viewed as the place where caring is possible. Thus, caring and not caring can be seen as opposite heads of the same coin. Just as there exists the possibility for psychological caregiving to occur, so too exists the possibility that it will not occur. In the stories presented in Chapter 1, staff had, at the moment of choice, acted in such a way that their patients' psychological needs were not fully realised. The nurses described had not seized all possibilities for delivering psychological care. Their explanations for their choices, and their personal experience in making them are, of course, unknown, but the negative effects of their choices are evident.

While there are always competing priorities, sometimes the decision about what must be attended to first (in the interests of preserving life and ensuring safety) is clear cut:

> You haven't got enough staff to talk to patients because you're doing the physical care needs, it's the first priority, do you suction somebody who's got a tracheotomy and is choking, whose sats [saturation of blood gases] are dropping, and if you don't care for that need, or you're neglecting that need, and you're talking to somebody who's upset because he's just found out he's got cancer, in the same bay across the way, and me personally, although I'm into psychological care . . . I'll maintain the person's airway.

However, in less life-threatening situations, staff need to find a way to weigh up the competing demands and reach a decision about what to attend to first. Often, when there are competing priorities for time and attention, psychological care is not seen as an 'important thing' and may be neglected: 'I think that some people are more in a rush sometimes, some people . . . don't think about the psychological needs, they just skip them and just do the important things and go'.

The further that nurses rise in the hierarchy, the more pressing the competing priorities become. It may be easier, then, for students to identify and use time to attend to psychological needs than for experienced staff: 'I've got a lot more time, because the [qualified] nurses have always got something to do on their mind'.

There is a general sense that psychological care will not happen automatically; it is a conscious, deliberate activity, and room must be made or identified for it, for example:

> With the practice here, with being on the ward, I've found that the physical needs, you know, the feeding and toileting, bed bathing, take priority now . . . but there is lots of room for psychological caregiving. They have a lot of anxieties and time has to be made.

> Even though you were busy, busy and I mean really busy, I always, always in a morning spent five or ten minutes with each patient, even if it was a patient that could do [everything] for themselves, totally independent, just give them that five minutes to say how they're feeling that morning, because it is really, really important.

> Rather than sitting at the nurses' desk, if you've got five minutes, you know, or gossiping with the other nurses, you'd go and spend five minutes with the patient.

Making the decision to prioritise psychological needs, however, sometimes brings its own challenges in busy clinical situations. Making room for patients to express their initial concerns and worries is sometimes seen as 'cruel' if there will be no time to follow up on these concerns or to give them full attention due to competing priorities, so sometimes the conscious decision is taken not to engage with psychological issues at all:

> I think sometimes, it sounds cruel, but not talking about it at all is better if you're busy, you've got to leave the patient, than opening up and acknowledging it, and then leaving them in mid flow and then not going back to them to finish that off, and I think that happens sometimes and it's wrong, but it happens due to other constraints.

The decision not to engage with patients' emotions at a 'caring moment' (Watson 1999) sometimes means that the moment for making a connection with the patient is lost:

> You . . . open up a bag of worms, and then you have to leave it. And the patient's there amid sort of emotions, I want to talk now, where are you, and you go in to the patient after, he's closed back up to you, he won't trust you again, because they trusted you with what they've said and you haven't had the time to listen to them so . . . I think sometimes that's why nurses keep things superficial, oh is your husband coming in to see you today, I bet you're missing him, and all this superficial stuff, skirting over the issues.

The importance of 'small acts'

What is important to recognise, though, is that in many cases, despite lack of time and competing priorities, psychological care can be delivered very quickly and effectively by small and apparently trivial actions: the 'little things' that contribute to the 'big picture'. These small acts may not be essential in the same way that some aspects of physical care are essential to survival. Nonetheless they are at least as important and contribute greatly to patients' sense of well-being:

> I then noticed some unopened cards. The patient brightened up and asked me to find his reading specs. I looked around, eventually finding his specs inside his wash bag. I left the patient happily reading his cards, now feeling happier and not neglected.

> Just sit and hold their hand, just while you're talking to them.

But it is easy to miss these little things that can make a big difference:

> Luckily the other staff member saw that the window across the room was open and the curtains had been drawn and were blowing, she went over and shut the window, whereby, the patient promptly went quiet and smiled at her.

The omission of small acts of caring can result in a sense of a general lack of care:

> We had a man who flew in from Tokyo to see his mum, complete with suitcases, and nobody offered him a drink, he was just left to go into his mum, and nobody bothered, and that man had just flown in from Tokyo . . . to me that is basic, because, you know, that comes first, I'd be devastated if I'd travelled all that way and not got a drink.

Little things, although recognised as having potentially large effects, are not always deemed to be legitimate parts of caregiving and are therefore not often documented, which diminishes their perceived importance:

You'd end up with care plans like 'such a body is upset, she's started worrying about her condition' . . . you can't write down 'hold her hand, make a cup of tea, give her ten minutes personal attention', can you? It's all the little things that would look ludicrous perhaps, written down . . . you can't possibly, you'd be documenting every working minute of the day.

We noted, in Chapter 1, the general consensus that caring comprises instrumental and expressive elements, and intuitively, caring for psychological needs would seem to be most closely aligned with the expressive elements of care rather than with the instrumental or practical, task-focused elements. However, from the quotations above, it seems that certain elements of psychological care could be considered as instrumental elements, in that they are practical tasks often with a physical care focus (such as making a cup of tea or closing a window). What seems to be important here is the intention behind the act, which in these instances was to enhance patients' well-being, and to produce a sense of safety, comfort, and control that extended beyond their needs for physical or instrumental care activities.

The notion of care delivered effectively through small acts is not extensively reported within the literature, although both Diekelmann (1993) and Hanson and Smith (1996) in studies of nursing students' experiences of caring by teachers, noted that influential caring interactions were often 'small acts that could go unnoticed' (Hanson and Smith 1996: 111). In terms of nursing practice, MacLeod's (1994) phenomenological study of nursing expertise suggested that the 'little things' that nurses do make a difference to individual patients because they are suffused with nursing knowledge and skill, but are largely hidden within the complexity of everyday nursing practice. Examples of such 'little things' in MacLeod's study were making a handle out of a bandage for a chest drain bottle in order that a patient could walk independently to the toilet, and repositioning a bath mat so that a patient felt safe to get out of the bath. Further, the notion of psychological care in practice being most effectively delivered through small acts is well illustrated by Wondrak's (1998) account of a patient with a prolonged high temperature. In this patient's description of his care experience, he identified three types of nurse: the techno-type, the care plan type, and the intuitive type. The intuitive type is the kind of nurse most able to have an empathic map of the patient's experience, and the nurse in this illustration helped him to sponge himself down to feel cooler, and replaced a plastic mattress cover with a cotton one. These were small acts primarily designed to improve the patient's physical health. However, the effect that they had was far-reaching in terms of the patient's overall sense of well-being. The patient felt reassured, safe and cared for.

Within the stories presented in Chapter 1, only small acts were needed to make a difference to the patients' experience. A few words of personal introduction, the offering of an explanation of delay, the positioning of the nurse call bell, for example, all small acts in themselves, but by their absence they had a profound effect on the patients' experience of care. Priest's (2001) study was permeated with examples of small acts, such as spending time to complete a crossword with a patient, or using a notebook to aid communication, all of which nurses identified as having significant effects upon their patients' psychological well-being. By their very nature, small acts are often invisible or pass unnoticed to the observer as exemplars of effective caring. When they occur, they are often taken for granted.

It is true that psychological care is often delivered through the medium of physical care, which facilitates the development of a relationship that forms the basis of psychological caregiving (Pegram 1992). James (1992) claimed that because they are the most visible components of care, physical tasks provide a timetable and a framework for care. Accepting physical caregiving as the medium through which psychological needs are addressed might, though, result in nurses overlooking psychological care needs at a time not designated for physical care. In order to safeguard against this it has been suggested that psychological care should be 'identified quite explicitly as a treatment and assigned to a designated member of the ward or clinic team' (Wilson-Barnett 1994: 25). In line with this, and suggesting that not all nurses are suitable for psychological care work, Nichols (1993) has proposed that a hospital ward should be able to draw upon a pool of interested and appropriately trained nurses, whose responsibilities would be to deal with the psychological care needs of patients arriving on the ward. In this way, attention to the psychological needs of all patients would be guaranteed. This at first seems incompatible with the contemporary focus on a holistic, individualised approach to care. However, it shares some similarities with the 'link nurse' role as operates in some health care settings, whereby individual nurses with a particular interest and training in, say, wound care or nutrition, adopt this as their focus within a ward team, and are responsible for advising and disseminating best practice within the team.

In reality, although the term 'psychological care' may be documented on care plans, in practice there is frequently little or no explanation of how, and by whom, that care is to be delivered (Wilkinson 1996). This may be because although psychological care is no less a part of nursing practice than physical care, as nurses become more experienced, psychological caregiving activities become 'second nature' and hard to recognise (Jost 1995). It may also be that nurses do not fully understand the nature or components of psychological care, nor how best to deliver it, perhaps because of shortcomings in educational preparation. A simple psychological care plan, which could accompany any physical care plan and which might ensure that patients' psychological needs are at least considered, is included in Chapter 5.

Action point

Reflect on your current or most recent clinical work.

Identify those aspects of your caring role that demonstrate attention to patients' psychological needs.

Having read this chapter, are there any things that you might now do differently?

Consequences of giving and receiving psychological care

The final component of the model of psychological care (Figure 4.3) to consider is the consequence of giving and receiving, on the part of the carer and the patient.

Consequences for patients

The consequences for patients of receiving timely and effective psychological care are that their psychological well-being is maintained or improved. Anxiety is reduced and they experience a feeling of safety and are empowered within the constraints of their illness. As one nurse noted: 'I think it is one of the most important [things], to reduce anxiety levels and hopefully reduce stress levels, but I think it's just giving them the time as well to express any problems they've got'.

However, if they do not receive adequate psychological care, they experience uncertainty, are not in control, and are anxious, as illustrated by a nurse who had personal experience of the lack of psychological care as a patient's relative:

> The day that my dad had his operation he went down to the surgical ward, and from suddenly having all the support we had absolutely nothing, because all that they knew was they had a man from theatre and the operation had gone well, and they ignored us. Nobody would tell us anything. And I actually told the staff how we felt, because we'd had so much, I don't know if they'd really protected us upstairs, because every day they were telling us how poorly he was, and then to suddenly come down here, all you're interested in is oh yes he's alright, and it was ever so hard, that was really, really hard.

Consequences for carers

As noted by Griffin (1983: 294), 'as a result of . . . caring a nurse may have an increased sense of personal worth'. When effective and timely psychological care has been delivered, it can be experienced as a pleasurable moment, in which a connection with the experience of the patient is felt, and one that brings personal reward:

> During the experience I felt a sense of doing something worthwhile and useful to the patient in a way that doing something like bandaging a leg or applying a dressing is seen as necessary to the patient's recovery. Little things (are) not really a necessity to the patient but in terms of personal pleasure it is worth a whole lot more.

> Patients' feedback, when they tell you you're going to be a good nurse . . . so you want to keep going, I mean you must be doing something right . . . it's job satisfaction. It feels good.

However, as well as being rewarding, the experience is personally demanding; hence the need for effective support and self care:

> When I've got two or three (terminally ill patients) that are actually coming up to the last, you know quite intensive nursing, it's very stressful, and I know I can tell I'm very stressed when I'm working, I'm more irritable, and I can't eat properly, I'm rushing around because I want to give them . . . the high level of care.

> Trying to be looking after the acute problems, and looking after these people who are distressed and wanting your attention, it's awful, because you feel as though you're saying to everybody, just a minute just a minute, and never really getting down to finding out what's wrong with that person and what's distressing them.

Consequently, as we have noted earlier in this chapter, nurses execute choice about whether or not they offer psychological care. Although sometimes not giving psychological care is due to a failure to identify need, sometimes it is a deliberate act of choice. The location of that choice varies; it may be attributed to external causes, such as the ward ethos:

> It's how the ward approaches it, I mean the surgical ward's main priority was get somebody from theatre, make sure their obs (observation of vital signs) and everything are alright, get them home for the next one to go in.

When psychological care is not delivered, whether due to external or internal reasons, the experience is of guilt and frustration:

> You're not caring, you're just providing, that's the best way of putting it.

> You feel very guilty . . . that you're not doing, providing that sort of input, but you know that you're always going to be disturbed and the patients, they need somebody that they know is going to give them some attention and support.

> When you develop that relationship with a patient, and talk very briefly, you can see they're upset, and it's very frustrating because you can't say well, stuff everything else that's going on, you need to talk. But sometimes again they've lost the moment by doing that.

In some cases the frustration turns to a sense of failure in the job and the experience of personal distress:

> I think that's what causes me a lot of psychological distress really, the fact that I don't feel that I'm providing the best care that I can, to people that are passing through our ward . . . When I can't carry that through I think that's when I get really, really dissatisfied with the job.

In describing an incident in which she was unable to identify the needs of a non-English speaking patient, one nurse commented:

> I found this particular incident rather distressing and upsetting for both the patient and myself. Psychologically I feel that this patient's needs are not being met because of the lack of communication with those around him . . . It is also extremely difficult to know what he may be thinking or feeling or even what his overall mental state is like. This was one experience, which I would not like to have again. It was not only infuriating for me, it was unbelievably frustrating.

Summary

In this chapter, we have traced the development of theories and models of psychological care, mostly from the nursing field, and noted that nurses are often viewed as the primary providers of psychological care (Nichols 1993). We have seen, too, that although psychological care should be an integral part of holistic care delivery, in reality it is often an added extra that is most likely to be provided through the medium of physical care delivery. Patients' requirements for psychological care are rarely documented on nursing care plans. It can, therefore, be easy for psychological needs to be overlooked. To enable us to fill in the gaps in documenting psychological care on a care plan, we explore both the 'core' elements of psychological care and some of the preconditions further in the next three chapters. Specifically, we explore the personal qualities, skills and knowledge needed to be an effective psychological caregiver.

5 Qualities for psychological care

Can I *be* in some way which will be perceived by the other person as trustworthy, as dependable or consistent in some deep sense?

(Carl Rogers 1958)

Introduction

In the quotation above, Carl Rogers seems to be asking whether there is a 'way of being' that will communicate a clear message to another person about his qualities and personality; in other words, what can another person expect of him if they enter into a relationship with him? In Chapter 4, we identified the core components of psychological caregiving, and some preconditions for delivering psychological care effectively. Amongst the preconditions identified was a set of personal qualities, and in this chapter, we explore the broad nature of 'personal qualities' before examining in more detail those that are thought to underpin effective psychological care, including self awareness, intuition, reflection, relationship building, and empathy. We draw particularly on Rogers' important work in explaining the concept of empathy.

What is a personal quality?

Action points

Write an advertisement offering yourself 'for sale' as a friend. Emphasise your best features and strengths. When you have finished, review your advertisement and identify the elements that you consider to be your 'personal qualities'.

Your advertisement may have contained a mixture of facts, such as 'young' or 'blonde'; practical attributes or interests, such as 'sporty' or 'musical'; and aspects of your personality such as 'outgoing' or 'calm'. Reflecting on these personal aspects or qualities, to what extent do you think they are inborn, and to what extent have they developed over time?

Psychologists and researchers disagree about the extent to which our 'personality' is a static entity and so part of us that it is unlikely to change over time. For example, if you describe yourself as 'shy', does this mean that you will always be shy, or only in certain situations? Can you teach yourself (or be taught) to be 'not shy', and if so, does that mean you have changed an aspect of your personality, or just your ability to manage your behaviour as required in certain situations?

There is some broad agreement that core personality dimensions are either inborn (genetically predetermined) or developed in early childhood, and once established, are stable and resistant to substantial change (Eysenck 2009), although of course personality will modify and develop as we grow and as we are exposed to new people and situations. It is also generally agreed that 'personality' is made up of a set of core traits or characteristics that distinguish humans from other animals and which make each human unique. These traits are thought to include openness, conscientiousness, extraversion, agreeableness, and neuroticism (McCrae and Costa 1987), on which each individual has a unique profile; in other words, your personality is a unique set of characteristics and qualities that make you different from every other human being in the world. It is likely that it is our personal qualities that enable us to use our skills effectively. In relation to caring, then, it may be that we can identify some core personality characteristics or qualities that will facilitate psychological caregiving, but which can also be developed and enhanced by training and experience.

Action point

Imagine that you have a personal problem or difficulty that you would like to talk over with a friend or family member. Who would you choose, and why?

It is likely that you included in your reasons things like 'I can trust that person'; 'they will keep my confidence', or 'they will listen to me and not judge me'. As we shall see, the reasons why we choose certain people to share our problems with or confide in are exactly the reasons why our patients choose (or don't choose) to open up to us. However, there is no one pre-scribed set of personal qualities upon which the ability to care for psychological needs depends. As one nurse in Priest's study (2001) commented:

> It's hard to define because it comes from something that's within, what makes people want to care for others in the first place, it's an emotion isn't it, what drives that person to want to be a nurse and what drives that person wanting to be a lawyer.

However, participants did feel that to a large extent, the appropriate personal qualities were either present or not within a carer, and that they were likely to have been present before entering the health care arena, as shown in the following interview extracts:

> It's more to do with the person's beliefs and attitudes even before they start nursing, because you can only shape attitudes and beliefs so far.

> Yes I think it's personal, how the person is generally, not just something that they've picked up on the wards because they've been there a long time.

> I think a lot of it is the personality of the nurse as well, I've got to be honest, that some nurses are better at talking to patients than others, some nurses prefer the management role.

While this does not mean that nurses who 'prefer the management role' do not possess the requisite personal qualities, there is a view that some nurses would never be good at psychological caregiving, as suggested in this extract from a focus group interview with student nurses:

Interviewer: What is it about them, then, that means they . . .
Student 1: Well they just come across abrupt, and they're only here for the money, and why should they be bothered, get on with it. There are nurses like that about.
Interviewer: Do you think they might have been caring once?
Student 2: Yes, possibly, like us idealistic students.

However, it is recognised that the demands of the job may in some way have contributed to the loss or suppression of the requisite qualities, and that this is a risk faced by all nurses.

What, then, are the personal qualities necessary for effective psychological caregiving? Priest's (2001) research revealed that possessing an intuitive nature is a helpful quality in identifying and responding to patients' psychological needs. Other qualities are self aware-ness, empathy, genuineness, and a non-judgmental approach. It is perhaps not surprising that these are thought by many to be some of the core characteristics of an effective counsellor. Carl Rogers, introduced in Chapter 2 and often seen as the 'father' of modern counselling, produced a set of core conditions that he deemed crucial to any effective helping relation-ship. The conditions include the counsellor (helper) being *congruent* in the relationship, having an *unconditional positive regard* for the client, having an *empathic understanding* of the client's internal frame of reference, and *communicating* to the client that empathic understanding and unconditional positive regard (Rogers 1957). These core conditions can be defined as in Figure 5.1.

We will explore the quality of empathy in more depth later in this chapter. As well as being necessary conditions for being an effective helper, Carl Rogers (1957) took the view that 'no other conditions are necessary. If these . . . conditions exist, and continue over a period of time, this is sufficient'. In other words, provided that a counsellor possessed these core conditions/qualities, then that in itself would be sufficient to be helpful in a counselling relationship, without the need for specific skills or techniques.

Congruence in the relationship: congruence can also be described as genuineness, openness or transparency; the helper does not pretend to be anything other than what he or she is, and tries to ensure that all forms of communication (spoken, non-verbal) are congruent with one another. Being congruent should help to ensure that we do not give conflicting messages.

Unconditional positive regard: this means that the helper views the client or patient 'with dignity' and values them 'as a worthwhile and positive human being' without any conditions being applied, such as expecting something back from the relationship (Burnard 2005: 102). Hence there is a genuine acceptance of and respect for another human being, simply because they are a human being, and not judging them for any behaviours, attitudes or opinions that we may find difficult or unacceptable.

Empathic understanding: often referred to simply as 'empathy'. This is the ability to see the world as the other person sees it, and convey this perceptual understanding back to the patient or client.

Figure 5.1 Core conditions for effective helping relationships (from Rogers 1957)

> **Reflection point**
>
> To what extent do you think that the core conditions are both necessary and sufficient to bring about helpful change in an interpersonal relationship? (It may help to think about – when patients/clients choose you to share a problem with, is it because of the sort of person you are, and the 'core conditions' you may possess, or because of your technical skills?)

Most people would agree that these conditions are necessary. As pointed out by Biley (2005), 'Nurses make a difference by simply being with patients and relatives during difficult times, by showing kindness and compassion, empathy and understanding' (Biley 2005: 18). However, not everyone would agree that the core conditions are sufficient in their own right. Some authors have been critical of Rogers' view in that it fails to take into account the wider physical and social environment and context in which an individual finds him or herself (Bach and Grant 2009), while others such as Egan (2001) (whose model is perhaps more focused on arriving at solutions than simply exploring the problem), feel that more specific techniques such as challenging and goal setting are also necessary to bring about therapeutic change. We discuss basic counselling skills further in Chapter 6, but for now we will begin by examining the personal quality of self awareness.

Self awareness

What does it mean to be self aware, and how do we become self aware? In developmental psychology terms, young babies are not thought to possess any real sense of themselves as individuals separate from those around them and caring for them. This awareness of themselves as separate and unique individuals begins to develop during infancy when they begin to recognise themselves, for example, when they look at themselves in a mirror wearing a hat, they touch the hat on their own head. From that time, the development of self and self identify develops apace until adolescence and early adulthood. We briefly introduced Erikson's theory of identity development in adolescence in Chapter 2; upon reaching adulthood most people have developed a clear idea of who they are as unique individuals: their key characteristics, strengths, and weaknesses. There are many aspects of ourselves about which we can be self aware: our thoughts, feelings, sensations, sexuality, spirituality, physical state, appearance, levels of knowledge, and our needs and wants (Burnard 2005). Arguably, in a caring profession, self awareness is critical and can be seen as the extent to which our view of who we are and what we are like, as carers, is in harmony with how others (those we are caring for) actually see us.

In 1955, Joseph Luft and Harry Ingham developed the Johari window to show different elements of awareness and ways in which self awareness can be increased in interactions with others. The model shows that there are normally elements of our personality that we are either unaware of, or that we *are* aware of but choose to keep hidden from others, perhaps because we are not so happy about these aspects. Figure 5.2, the Johari window, is a diagrammatic representation of these elements.

Arguably, without knowing how we function ourselves when in difficulty or under stress, we will find it difficult to imagine how others might feel in similar situations. So to be self

Public Self (known to ourselves and others)	**Blind Self** (known to others but not to us)
Hidden (Private) Self (known to us but not to others)	**Unknown Self** (not known to us or others)

Figure 5.2 The Johari window

(from Luft and Ingham 1955)

aware is to be sensitive to the needs of others. It is important, too, that as well as recognising our positive traits, we recognise and own our biases, prejudices and stereotyped beliefs and the ways in which these might impact on our care delivery (McCabe and Timmins 2006). Figure 5.3 shows that if we listen to and respond to feedback from others, we will learn more about ourselves, and therefore have less within us that is 'blind'.

Self awareness is particularly relevant in nursing and health care at the time when we are making decisions about how to respond to our patients' needs. Priest's (2001, 2006) study showed that nurses recognise that there is always the possibility for psychological care, but that they then make a choice about whether or not to respond to patients' psychological needs. Several other concepts are linked to self awareness. These are self disclosure, self acceptance, and self care.

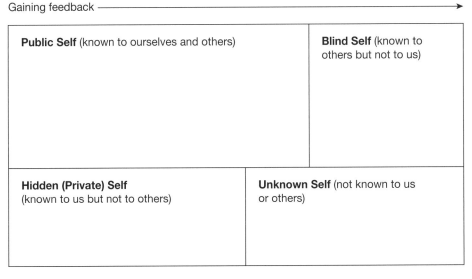

Figure 5.3 Increasing self awareness

(from Luft and Ingham 1955)

Self disclosure

Self disclosure is a deliberate act of sharing aspects of ourselves with other people so that they get to know us better. The more we disclose, the less of ourselves remains hidden, as we can see in the third version of the Johari window (Figure 5.4).

Self disclosure is important in the development and maintenance of successful inter-personal relationships, but needs to be reciprocal. Imagine that you have just shared some very personal information with a friend, revealing some of your deeply held worries. In return, you might reasonably expect your friend to respond by sharing some of his or her views and feelings, to help you to feel that you are not alone or different, and that your friend feels sufficiently comfortable and secure with you to reciprocate. This reciprocation relies on mutual trust. However, in professional caring relationships, such mutuality would not be expected, so how does self disclosure fit into the professional caring arena?

Reflection point

To what extent do you think that self disclosure is a) necessary and b) possible within professional caring relationships?

You may have thought that it is inappropriate to share much personal information within a professional caring context. After all, we do not enter into personal relationships with our patients, and there is no expectation or requirement that we should share our innermost secrets with those we are caring for, nor that we should disclose personal information that might identify, for example, exactly where we live. Most of us, after all, wish to maintain a clear boundary between our personal and professional lives. However, unless we self disclose to some extent, the less other people will get to know us, and the more difficult it will be to

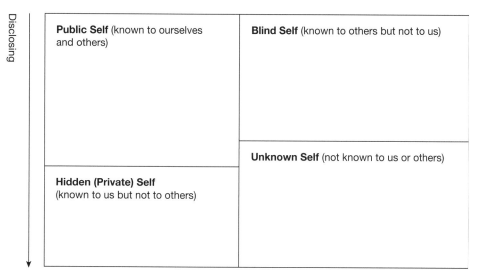

Figure 5.4 Increasing self disclosure

(from Luft and Ingham 1955)

make meaningful interpersonal relationships, which as we shall discover are fundamental for effective psychological care. You might like to try the following exercise to assess your own self disclosure behaviour and preferences, and to consider how these operate within your own clinical practice.

Action points

Write a list of 10 statements that best describe you, including the points that you consider to be positive and those you are less proud of.

Which of these statements would you be willing to share with a close friend?

Which, if any, would you be willing to share with a patient?

Consider the reasons for any differences.

Self acceptance

Closely linked with self disclosure is the concept of self acceptance. Accepting ourselves for who we are, with all our faults, is also a vital skill for establishing and maintaining relationships. The more aspects of ourselves we find difficult to like or accept, the less of ourselves we will wish to disclose to others. Why does this matter? Clearly the less we disclose, the less other people will get to know us. If they don't get to know us they can't accept us. This can become something of a vicious circle, because we will pick up that we are not accepted, which will in turn reinforce our own lack of self acceptance.

Self care

One other area in which it is particularly important to be self aware, when caring for others, is in identifying the need for support from others and for self care. We noted, in Chapter 4, that self care was a central component of Nichols' (1993) psychological care scheme. Attending to patients' psychological needs will place emotional demands upon carers, who may in turn experience anxiety and conflict if they feel unable to resolve patients' difficulties. So being self aware will enable us to monitor our stress levels and coping strategies and know when to seek support or help. Eventually, unless carers feel in some way cared for themselves, they will be unable to care for others (Grigsby and Megel 1995), so a supportive framework is required (Swanwick and Barlow 1994).

Reflection point

Do you feel cared for at work? What support strategies are in place in your workplace?

Effective teamwork and formal clinical supervision may be ways in which nurses and other care staff can receive support and comfort in their caring activities, and Nichols (2003) emphasised that psychological care cannot be delivered in an environment that did not make provision for the support of those providing that care. Furthermore, Nichols (1993) recognised that we should view seeking support not just as desirable, but also as a major professional responsibility. However, it has to be acknowledged that few clinical environments provide a structured system of staff support or clinical supervision. While long recognised as an important element of mental health nursing practice, clinical psychology, social work and counselling, the widespread adoption of clinical supervision in general nursing settings has been slower, although its implementation is gathering momentum (Heath and Freshwater 2000). Without appropriate supervision, nurses' reflective abilities will be hampered, and this will in turn hamper the provision of psychological care. It is also evident that nurses and other front line care staff are not good at caring for themselves or each other (Priest 2002; Sourial 1997). Without this, the effective provision of psychological care may remain an elusive ideal. We explore barriers to psychological care delivery further within Chapter 9, but for now, we move on to examine the quality of intuition.

Intuition

Intuition is sometimes thought of as having a 'sixth sense' or a 'gut instinct' that helps us to know what is happening for another person and perhaps how to respond appropriately. To a certain extent, intuition must be present in order for carers to tap into their patients' experience, and to identify and respond to patients' psychological needs. It refers to 'understanding without a rationale' (Benner and Tanner 1987), or 'knowledge and insights that arrive independently of the senses' (Burnard 2005: 72), and provides us with a different form of 'evidence' about how someone is feeling and what they need from that based on observations, objective measurements, logic and reason. Intuition has long been considered an important element in decision making in professional practice (e.g. Benner 1984, Greenwood and King 1995, King and Appleton 1997), although we might sometimes reject our intuitive decisions on the basis that we cannot trust our intuitions to be right (Burnard 2005).

Patricia Benner's (1984) important study of the ways in which nurses move from the position of complete beginner to experienced practitioner distinguished between the novice, who might possess the 'knowing that' of an activity, attained through context-free classroom leaning, and the expert, who is likely to possess know-how, or knowledge attained through practical, in-context experience, intuition and perceptual acuity, coupled with the flexibility to apply this know-how in a range of contexts. Priest's (2001) study of psychological care confirmed that expert nurses could not explain their abilities by cognitive knowledge alone; rather they placed heavy emphasis on intuition arising out of their experiences. The constant need to 'have your wits about you' and to pick up on cues was expressed.

> I tend just to go by my instincts how I feel the patient is, whether I feel we're brewing up for a crisis because they can't cope, and then intervene if I feel it's necessary . . . I think just generally you can pick up vibes.

The experienced nurses were clear that an intuitive ability was a pre-requisite for effective psychological caregiving:

> Nobody can tell you what it's about, what caring's about, or what do you mean by psychological care, it's something you sort of, I don't know, nursing intuition, I don't know, it's something from within . . . it's a much overlooked aspect of care, is nursing

intuition. Not only because it's difficult to validate, not much research has been done into it, and it's something about a gut reaction, what a nurse feels, and it's something you can't quantify, and it's something that's very esoterical [*sic*].

Although intuition is often considered part of expert practice, acquired through years of knowledge and experience (Taylor 2000), in this study (Priest 1999) beginning student nurses were clear that they used intuitive ability within their practice, and stressed the importance of intuition in developing their ability to give psychological care. In contrast to Benner's suggestion, they did not appear to have had to learn general rules before being able to apply them to different care situations. As one student nurse in this study, describing her ability to pick up cues from her patients about their psychological needs, commented: 'Nine times out of ten I've been right . . . but I don't know whether it's intuition, I don't know, I just seem to be able to'. And as another student commented: 'There's no text books, there's no theories, it's just a gut instinct'.

In other words, these students seem to have been able to operate from a 'knowing how' position even though they were relatively inexperienced. So perhaps intuition is not the exclusive province of the expert and may therefore be something that new entrants bring with them into the caring professions. This might support the idea that intuition is an innate personal quality, or perhaps it is a good intuitive sense that leads people to enter the caring professions in the first place.

Reflection

In order to develop our intuitive ability, we must have the ability to reflect on our actions and alter them appropriately if required. Increasingly, health care training programmes have as one of their aims the development of reflective practitioners. This is because, it could be argued, reflection involves making sense of experiences so as to learn from them; thus learning cannot take place without reflection. Indeed, this book includes 'action point' and 'reflection point' exercises which ask the reader to stop and think about a specific situation or experience and make personal sense of it, in order to develop learning. Taylor (2005: 8) defines reflection, in relation to health care practice, as 'throwing back thoughts and memories, in cognitive acts such as thinking, contemplation, meditation, and any other form of attentive consideration, in order to make sense of them, and to make contextually appropriate changes if they are required'.

Much of our contemporary understanding of reflection comes from the work of Donald Schön, a philosopher and organisational researcher, who among other things was interested in exploring professionals' ability to 'think on their feet'. In 1991, he published *The Reflective Practitioner* in which he distinguished between reflection 'on action' and reflection 'in action', both of which are highly relevant in health care practice. Reflection on action implies that we must be able to think about our interventions and care after the event; be able to judge the efficacy of our actions and care; and plan different future strategies if necessary. Discussions with supervisors, teachers, and colleagues on events and experiences after they have happened can often serve to facilitate such reflections on action.

On the other hand, reflection in action means that we must also be able to reflect on interventions and interactions, and adjust them, as they are happening – the 'thinking on your feet' quality that is so often an integral part of caring practice. Reflecting in action can be difficult as the practitioner may have to respond quickly in some care settings. As one nurse commented:

At first . . . you think 'oh, why did I do that', but then when you get more experience you learn to think about something while you're doing it and you see yourself getting better at what you do . . . You think maybe that wasn't quite so good, try and do it better next time.

Reflective practice is often illustrated as a 'cycle'; such as the experiential learning cycle proposed by Kolb (1984) and illustrated by Gibbs and Priest (2009), which includes the phases of:

- **Concrete experience**, in which learners involve themselves fully, openly, and without bias in new experiences.
- **Reflective observation**, in which learners are encouraged to step out of 'doing' and into reflecting on and analysing their experience from many perspectives, and sharing their thoughts with others.
- **Abstract conceptualisation**, in which learners think more deeply and attempt to interpret, understand and make links and comparisons between the experience and what they already know. At this point, they often seek to take control of their own learning.
- **Active experimentation**, in which they consider how they are going to put into practice what they have learnt and understood, make decisions and solve problems, and predict what will happen next. It is during this final stage where the student needs to see how their learning is useful.

This last stage leads back to new concrete experiences which will in turn provide material for further reflection.

Reflection point

Think back to when you were last consciously aware of 'reflecting' on your practice and changing something as a result. Can you identify the stages of Kolb's cycle within this experience?

In relation to psychological care, an example using Kolb's model might be as in Figure 5.5.

An alternative model of reflective practice is provided by Gibbs (1988) in relation to a personally experienced event (such an event is often referred to as a 'critical incident'). While it helps to reflect 'on action', the first stage encourages us to recreate the situation mentally as though it was happening now, so such an exercise may also help us to develop our 'reflection in action' abilities. A summary of Gibbs' model is shown in Figure 5.6.

Of course, the distinction between 'personal quality' and 'skill' is not clear-cut in relation to reflection, and while we have written about it here as though it were an intrinsic quality that one either possesses or does not, the fact that reflection is in itself a device to enhance learning must mean that it is something that can be learned and developed through observation, direct teaching, using reflective models to facilitate the process, and above all, practice. The same is true of the next personal quality that we will highlight: making relationships.

A nurse has the **concrete experience** of supporting a patient who has just received the news that her breast cancer has returned and that her future health and life expectancy are compromised. The nurse notes her own responses using **reflective observation** ('I don't know enough about this to give the correct information'; 'I feel so sorry for her'; 'I don't know what to say'). She then, in the process of **abstract conceptualisation,** recognises that to give incorrect information will not be helpful to her patient, and neither will feeling sorry for her or avoiding the situation altogether. She also recognises that being honest about her lack of knowledge, and willingness to find out, might be more helpful than doing and saying nothing. Finally, using **active experimentation,** she tells her patient honestly that she doesn't know what this might mean, and that she will seek further information from the medical consultant. She makes a time to return and spend some time with the patient, giving her the opportunity to discuss her feelings and fears.

Figure 5.5 Reflecting on experiences to enhance learning

Description: What happened?
Feelings: What did I think and how did I feel at the time?
Evaluation: What was good and what was bad about what I did?
Analysis: What sense did I make of this situation?
Conclusion: What else could I have done?
Action: What would I do differently if the situation arose again?

Figure 5.6 Reflective cycle (Gibbs 1988)

Action point

Identify a recent 'critical incident' in your caring activities. Using the steps above, reflect on this incident.

Making relationships

Writing about bringing about personality change in another individual, Carl Rogers (1957) suggested that 'a minimal relationship, a psychological contact, must exist'. While our endeavour as nurses and carers of physically ill people is not about producing 'personality change', nonetheless there is evidence to suggest that to be effective in any caring encounter, at least a rudimentary interpersonal relationship must be present. The need for the formation and maintenance of a relationship between nurse and patient in order for psychological caregiving to occur has previously been identified. Tanner, Benner, Chesla, and Gordon (1993) stressed the importance of knowing the patient in terms of his/her typical patterns of responses and knowing the patient as a person. The presence of a therapeutic relationship was argued as a precondition of caring by Hyland and Donaldson (1989). Rimon (1979), too, noted that through demonstrating an ability and willingness to listen, nurses would be able to build interpersonal relationships with their patients. However, it should be noted that the setting in which Rimon made this conclusion was rehabilitation, in which it might be expected that time would be available to develop meaningful interpersonal relationships. More recently, Barker (2003) has commented that the purpose of nursing is 'to come to know patients as human beings in difficulty' and that the therapeutic relationship is 'the crux of clinical nursing', and 'the cornerstone of nursing practice'.

As with intuition and reflection, however, it is quite difficult to decide whether the ability to form, maintain, and ultimately end a relationship with a patient is in fact a personal quality, or if it is more of a skill that can be learned. We have decided, perhaps arbitrarily, to consider it here as a personal quality, given that it is something that some people find relatively easy and others find extremely difficult, and that these differences can often be observed in even very young children. This is not to say that those who find relationship building difficult can never be good at psychological care. As we shall see, it is often only necessary for a very brief and transient relationship to have been formed; brief eye contact, perhaps, or the exchange of a smile, but enough to be able to say 'I have acknowledged your presence as a fellow human being, and you have acknowledged mine; therefore we are in a relationship with one another'.

Reflection point

How would you define a 'relationship' (as it exists between two people)?

What are the characteristics of an effective interpersonal relationship?

To what extent are these characteristics present in nurse/carer–patient interactions?

Attree (2001) showed that patients and relatives defined 'good care' in nursing as something provided through the presence of a caring relationship by staff. Within this caring relationship, patients are known as people; there is a bond or rapport; there is open communication and information sharing; there is kindness, concern, compassion, and sensitivity on the part of the nurse; the nurse is available and accessible; and takes and spends time with the patient. Reynolds and Scott (2000: 228) summarised the importance of a relationship underpinning effective nursing assessment: 'unless clients are able to trust nurses in an open two-way relationship, it is unlikely that nurses will be able to assess accurately the needs and problems of their clients from a client centred viewpoint'. Look back at your reflections on the characteristics of an effective relationship. Did any of these elements feature? Did you conclude that the fundamental characteristics of a relationship do exist in nurse/carer–patient interactions?

You might also have considered that patients may not expect or require an interpersonal relationship with their nurses (Muxlow 1995, Salvage 1990). In Ersser's (1990) study exploring how nursing affected patients' welfare, for example, a relationship was not often cited as a feature of a beneficial nurse–patient interaction. In some studies, brief interactions would be unlikely to be deemed relationships. Holyoake (1997), for example, found that nurses considered relationships to be something in which multiple interactions took place. Whether or not patients expect or require an interpersonal relationship with their nurses, findings of Priest's (2001) study make clear that the existence of a relationship, no matter how brief or how transient, was of importance in determining the provision or otherwise of psychological care. A relationship was deemed to have been made, for example, when even a brief moment of eye-to-eye contact or small piece of verbal exchange had taken place. With no relationship in place, the provision of psychological care was seen as unlikely if not impossible. Participants did not specify the precise form of the relationship that was needed to facilitate psychological caregiving, although the implication was that even a brief interaction facilitated a 'connection' with the patient (Morse 1991).

So what does this mean in practice? Often, the establishment of a relationship between carer and patient starts with simply 'opening a door' to communication, as shown by the quotations from nurses below:

> I generally go in and just chat to them. I don't tend to just ask too many specific questions at first, just to get, make them feel at ease with me . . . make them feel comfortable and try to get their trust.

> When I assess my patients I always pull the curtains round anyway and sit with them for a good twenty minutes just chatting about, you know, the weather, sometimes, and if they've got anything to say it'll normally come out in the conversation as the time goes on rather that just running round and saying quickly let me check your pulse right away, let me take your blood pressure.

Opening the door in this way facilitates the development of a relationship at a later time; in other words, the door is 'left open':

> I've found that to go over and introduce myself and just say, I'm one of your team nurses . . . if you want me just give me a shout, and I'll always tell them my name and I'll always say, if you want anything, just give me a shout, and that's your opening then . . . for that person will say oh she's really nice, dead approachable, whatever, and maybe I might, you know, and at a later date that gives you something to fall back on and they'll say oh yes she seems all right, I'll just call her over and have a word and they will spend five or ten minutes talking to you.

> I was pleased to be of service. If I had not offered my services to this mother at the beginning of the day, she may have felt staff were too busy to ask for help herself. My initial approach opened a pathway to easy communication.

If doors are left open but subsequently closed, the consequences can be detrimental to future psychological caregiving:

> I think we empower the patients quite a bit with the information giving that we're doing, and I think it gives the patients quite a bit of control if we say we're going to come back in ten minutes because we normally always do, and if we don't come back then they're not going to trust us the next time to come back.

Hildegard Peplau (1952) was a nurse theorist who introduced the concept of interpersonal relations as the basis for studying and practising nursing. She considered that the successful formation, maintenance, and termination of relationships between nurses and patients was the distinctive contribution that nursing could make to health care. Peplau went so far as to say that an effective nurse–patient relationship could transform symptom-bound anxiety into problem-solving energy. Although her model is of particular relevance in mental health nursing contexts, it has been considered by many to offer a useful framework for understanding the importance of interpersonal relationships in general nursing contexts. Figure 5.7 summarises Peplau's model.

According to Peplau, the therapeutic relationship progresses through a number of phases, as outlined in Figure 5.8, although in practice these phases often overlap.

The basic concepts within Peplau's model are anxiety and communication. In this context, anxiety is seen as a productive energy source in health, necessary for biological and emotional growth, but which becomes 'bound' in illness, affecting the patient's ability to function effectively and producing non-healthy symptoms. During the orientation phase, at the commencement of the relationship, patients experience a need and seek help; in response, nurses help patients to clarify their difficulties and determine their need for help. The identification phase is the time for establishing good interpersonal communication, such that patients accept the nurse as a helpful partner in their care; exploration of feelings is encouraged during this phase, and a plan of care is formulated. In the exploitation or working phase, the aim is to alleviate the patient's anxiety and transfer power from the nurse back to the patient. This might, for example, involve the nurse in using counselling skills (see Chapter 6). In the resolution phase, a mutual withdrawing from the relationship takes place and the success of the relationship in alleviating the patient's anxieties is evaluated.

To facilitate progression through these phases of the therapeutic relationship, Peplau believed that nurses need to adopt and move between a number of different yet overlapping roles, as listed in Figure 5.9.

At the initial stage of a relationship, neither party knows the other; hence they are strangers to one another. During this stage, the nurse's role is to accept the patient, to be non-judgemental and to establish trust. As a resource person, the nurse's role is to communicate relevant knowledge, skills and experience. As a teacher, the nurse gives the patient instructions and provides information. As a leader, the nurse's role is to lead the patient towards achieving their goals. As a surrogate, the nurse can 'stand in' for the patient or other people in the patient's life, and may, for example, act as an advocate in speaking up for the patient about what treatment he or she wants to undertake. As a counsellor, the nurse helps the patient to

---

- The nurse and the patient participate in the relationship
- The relationship itself can be therapeutic; that is, the relationship is a form of treatment
- It provides the basis for nursing assessment
- It enables patients to learn more satisfactory and productive patterns of behaviour
- It reduces anxiety

Figure 5.7 Principles of Peplau's model of interpersonal relationships in nursing

---

- Orientation phase
- Identification phase
- Exploitation or working phase
- Resolution phase
- Termination phase

Figure 5.8 Phases of the therapeutic relationship (Peplau)

- Stranger
- Resource person
- Teacher
- Leader
- Surrogate
- Counsellor

Figure 5.9 Roles in the therapeutic relationship (Peplau)

discuss and face the feelings which the illness experience is generating. These roles operate with the overall goal of anxiety reduction.

Peplau's model has been criticised in that with its focus on interpersonal relationships it has failed adequately to take into account wider social systems and their influence on patients' problems. Clearly, a person's psychological state in illness will be influenced by external social and environmental factors, which would need to be considered by a nurse planning and delivering care. Despite this criticism, the fact that the aims of intervention within Peplau's model are the nurse–patient relationship and the alleviation of anxiety means that the model should be able to facilitate the identification of and care for psychological needs. As we will discover, any meaningful relationship depends for its existence upon at least a degree of empathy with the other person's situation or perspective. Thus a nurse's efforts to establish such a relationship would require him or her to try to understand the patient's thoughts, feelings and experiences, and thereby tap into psychological needs. It is easy to dismiss the goal of anxiety reduction as of low priority when compared with the need to ensure physiological integrity. Yet if anxiety is seen as the result of inability to meet a goal of any kind, then the relevance of anxiety reduction as the primary focus of nursing and caring becomes more apparent. Peplau's premise was that relationships form the basis for providing total physical care, emotional support and health education through the illness experience (Arnold 1999). Perhaps, then, Peplau's (1952) model should be reconsidered as an appropriate framework for holistic nursing care in physical illness.

Reflection point

What might be the difficulties in using relationships as the basis for good psychological care?

Clearly, some patients may have difficulties in trusting their carer enough to enter into a relationship with them. Maintaining relationships may be difficult, especially if there is a history of disruptive relationships in the past. There may be difficulties (on either side) of maintaining and respecting the professional boundaries and power differentials that must exist that make professional relationships different from personal relationships (we would not, for example, exchange mobile phone numbers with our patients, while this would be a very normal thing to do within the context of a new friendship). Ending relationships can be difficult, and arguably, if a therapeutic relationship is central to psychological caregiving, what happens when it is discontinued at the point of discharge? Are we encouraging dependency and setting up our patients for an avoidable experience of loss in the future? Equally, some carers may find it difficult to adopt the principle of having 'unconditional positive regard' for all their patients, regardless of their personal circumstance or characteristics. We don't instantly like every person we meet, and often the behaviours that they engage in frankly make it unlikely that we ever would enter into a relationship with them. So we are not always going to find it easy to have that non-judgmental acceptance of all our patients, no matter how professionally we try to behave. We explore the concepts of unconditional positive regard and a non-judgmental stance further in Chapter 6.

There are more practical challenges in care settings where the development of a meaningful interpersonal relationship is a difficult aim. Such settings might include intensive care or care of older people, where communication might be hampered by sensory or cognitive impairment, and settings where there is a very rapid patient turnover, such as in medical assessment units or emergency departments. Nichols (1993) did, in fact, acknowledge that his model of psychological care, in which a working interpersonal relationship was inherent, was perhaps easier to execute in a relatively 'long-stay' area such as renal care than in areas where rapid patient turnover might hinder the development of meaningful interpersonal relationships.

Despite these challenges, relationship building remains the foundation upon which identifying and responding to psychological needs are built. In Priest's study, the existence of a relationship, no matter how brief or how transient, was found to be of importance in determining the provision or otherwise of psychological care. Relationship building starts with carers making the first move, introducing themselves and communicating availability and openness through good eye contact, smiling, and being courteous, respectful and tactful. The aim is to enable patients to feel comfortable in our presence, and we may begin with superficial social conversation. We leave the door open for future communication. Patients may choose not to enter into the relationship at once, but will store up their impressions of these initial overtures for later use, which will guard against perceptions of us as being 'too busy' for them. Initial overtures facilitate pathways to easy communication later; they know us by name and can feel sufficient trust and security to express emotions and believe they will be listened to. The consequences of establishing such relationships are that the patient feels understood and valued as an individual, less isolated in an unfamiliar world and better able to maintain independence within the limitations of physical illness. Having trust that a particular individual will meet their needs provides them with some control at an otherwise out-of-control time.

With no relationship in place, the provision of psychological care is unlikely if not impossible. This might, then, facilitate a move towards what Nolan, Keady and Aveyard (2001) have described as 'the next logical step': relationship-centred care, in which the centrality of relationships in health care is not only affirmed but also promoted through the education of health care professionals.

Empathy

Finally, in our consideration of personal qualities that underpin psychological care, we turn our attention to empathy. Priest's research suggested that a pre-requisite personal quality for psychological caregiving is the ability to empathise; that is, to sense or have an 'empathic map' of the reality and experience of being a patient and its challenges and difficulties. As with Carl Rogers, Reynolds and Scott (2000) describe empathy as a core characteristic of a helping relationship, and one that has two components, the first of which is the ability to perceive the other person's feelings and make some sense out of that perception. However, it is not enough simply to have this understanding of what it might be like to be the patient at that time; it is equally important that we communicate this understanding of their 'feelings and attached meanings' to the patient, both verbally and non-verbally so that first, they feel understood, and second, they have the opportunity to correct us if we have gained an inaccurate sense of what they are feeling and needing. So what is empathy? Reynolds and Scott note that it has been defined in at least three different ways: as a behaviour; as a personality dimension or personal quality; and as an experienced emotion. Kunyk and Olson (2000) conducted a concept analysis of empathy and identified five different ways in which it could be conceptualised: as a human trait; as a professional state; as a communication process; as caring; and as a special relationship.

It is important, here, to make a distinction between the related concepts 'sympathy' and 'empathy'. The simplest way of explaining the distinction is to say that sympathy is imagining what we might feel like if we were in the same position as the patient. While sympathy in itself is not wrong, there is always the danger that if we dwell too deeply on how *we* might feel if we were in pain, or frightened of a procedure, or facing a poor prognosis, we might become engulfed in our own emotions and therefore less able to respond to the patient's emotions.

Empathy, on the other hand, takes the focus away from us and moves it onto them – trying to imagine how the patient actually feels in their situation; seeing the world through their eyes rather than our own. Of course it is never possible to enter the inner world of another person completely, but empathy is an attempt to get as close to that reality as possible. Sometimes empathy is described as having an 'as if' quality: trying to sense experiences and emotions 'as if' we were the patient (Rogers 1957). This is a subtle but important distinction from sensing how our own experiences and emotions might be in the same situation.

Reynolds and Scott (2000: 231) suggest that empathy in nursing can:

- enable nurses to create a climate of trust and establish what patients perceive they need;
- enable nurses to understand the origins and purpose of patients' responses to health problems;
- facilitate positive health outcomes such as the reduction of physiological distress, anxiety and depression.

Communicating empathy

We have already noted, however, that it is not enough simply to 'pick up' on patients' emotions and needs. Unless we communicate to them that we have sensed how they are feeling, they will have no sense of being heard or understood. So how do we communicate empathy? Sometimes it is enough to do this non-verbally, without even saying anything, for example by sitting at the same level as the patient; leaning towards them; making eye contact; mirroring their posture; sharing their silence; and perhaps using touch if appropriate. All of these actions say to the patient 'I'm here, I'm with you, I'm trying to get closer to you,' and are simple yet powerful ways of communicating empathy. If we wish to use words, then often simply repeating some of what the patient is saying to us, perhaps in our own words (paraphrasing), and perhaps in a questioning tone, demonstrates that we are listening and really trying to get close to the things that are important to them. Taking this one step further, we might observe the patient's body language and facial expressions to infer what they might be feeling, such as anger or fear, and reflect back what we have picked up, for example, by saying 'I sense from the way you are sitting/lying/looking that you might be feeling (for example, 'angry') right now. Is that right?' While we are going beyond the patient's words here, we are showing that we are really trying to see things from their point of view, while at the same time, allowing for them to correct our assumptions if we are wrong.

We are once again, perhaps, moving beyond 'personal qualities' and into the realm of 'interpersonal skills' (for example, paraphrasing and reflecting back are key skills in counselling), and in reality the division between qualities and skills is often not clear cut. For example, in Burnard's (1998) study in which student nurses were asked to identify the important personal qualities of a counsellor, a majority identified 'being a good listener' as a personal quality rather than a skill. Similarly, there is considerable debate about whether empathy is something inborn or whether we can learn to become empathic (or more empathic). How we define and understand empathy will influence how we become empathic. For example, if it is a behaviour, we could learn it by observing, practising, and gaining feedback on our performance of showing empathy. If it is a personal quality or an experienced emotion, then perhaps we have less control over our empathic abilities: we either have them or we do not.

Certainly it is possible to experience and communicate empathy at a number of levels (and indeed, not to communicate it at all). Carkhuff (1969) has illustrated this as 'levels of empathy', as shown in Figure 5.10.

It is important to note that Level 4 and 5 responses, while expressing 'deeper' levels of empathy, are not necessarily always 'good' empathic responses, especially if they make too many unfounded assumptions about what the other person is experiencing. In most cases in everyday caring practice, a Level 3 response is the most appropriate.

·	**Level 1**	Neither feelings nor content are acknowledged.
·	**Level 2**	Some slight reflection of either feelings or content.
·	**Level 3**	Both feelings and content are accurately reflected.
·	**Levels 4–5**	Feelings and/or content are acknowledged before the client has spoken of them or is fully aware of them.

Figure 5.10 Levels of empathy (from Carkhuff 1969)

Action point

Try to match the responses to the scenario below to the appropriate level of empathy as described by Carkhuff (suggested answers at the end of this chapter):

When you arrive on duty for your afternoon nursing shift, you notice Mrs Jones lying on her bed in a curled up position, with her face turned to the wall, and with tears running down her face. You go over to her bed and ask her how she is; she says she is upset because none of her family is able to visit today. You respond by saying:

1   Oh, well, never mind, I'm sure they will be along tomorrow.

2   Oh I'm so sorry they can't get in today; I imagine you're feeling really sad about that.
3   Gosh you must be feeling cold lying on top of your bed; shall I get you a blanket?
4   You must be feeling totally abandoned by your family and feel angry that they haven't bothered to come to see you.
5   Oh I'm sorry to hear that; I expect you miss them a lot while you're in hospital.

Unfortunately, it has been shown in numerous studies across different health care professions that health care staff, including nurses, do not show much empathy to patients and therefore probably operate at Level 1 or 2 for much of the time (see for example, Reynolds and Scott 2000). As a consequence, there can be unfavourable health outcomes if patients feel they have not been properly understood. Failure to understand their needs may result in nurses failing to provide important information or emotional support (Reynolds and Scott 2000), which in turn can lead to increased distress.

A consideration of empathy raises many questions. For example, can empathy be taught? To know whether it can be taught, we would need to have an effective way of measuring it so that the effects of any change following training could be demonstrated. A second key question is, can we empathise with everyone? Is it easier to empathise with someone whose situation or experience we are familiar with? If so, what would that mean (for example), for a 20-year-old physically fit and active female student physiotherapist working with a 40-year-old man who has just lost a leg in a motor cycling accident, and who can no longer play the competitive golf that he so loves? Clearly, we cannot have experienced every situation that our patients will present us with, nor do we often share their unique package of background, culture, age, and gender.

The critical factors, here, are first that empathy is about the other person's experience rather than how we might feel in the same situation, but second, that empathy is directed more towards the *emotion* underpinning an experience than towards the experience itself. Because we are all human and have experienced the full range of human emotions in our own lives, we can sense what it might be like for the other person. So, for example, the physiotherapy student above might draw upon her own experiences of having lost something precious to her (a broken relationship, or a family bereavement, for example) in tapping into the sadness and anger that her patient might be experiencing. In Chapter 6 we consider emotional care in more detail.

Summary

In this chapter, we have explored a number of personal qualities that are thought to underpin effective caring, and specifically, psychological caregiving. We have repeatedly noted that distinguishing personal qualities from caring skills is not easy and that sometimes the distinction is purely a matter of personal perspective. In the following chapter, we move on to consider the range of interpersonal skills that underpin professional psychological caregiving, taking note that the personal qualities we have explored are often themselves prerequisites for the development of such skills. Perhaps we must conclude, as Burnard (1998) did, that personal qualities are mediated through the demonstration of specific skills and that teasing out the distinction between the two is difficult if not impossible.

Suggested answers to action point (on pages 86–7)

1   This is a Level 2 response in which a minimal response to the content of Mrs Jones's message has been made, but there is no attempt to identify or communicate the perceived underpinning emotion.

2   This is a good Level 3 response; the message has been heard clearly and a real attempt is made to identify and communicate the emotion that Mrs Jones might be feeling.

3   This is a poor Level 1 response; neither the message nor the underpinning emotion has been addressed. Rather, the nurse tries to change the subject and avoid the issue altogether.

4   While both content and emotion have been identified, this response goes far beyond what Mrs Jones is expressing, and interpretations are made (feeling abandoned and angry) that cannot be assumed either by what she has said or by how she appears. Therefore this is a Level 4 or 5 response.

5   This is a reasonable Level 2 response; the content is acknowledged and there is an attempt at acknowledging the feeling by picking up that Mrs Jones might be 'missing' her family, but the underpinning emotion is not explored.

6 Skills for psychological care

Keep it simple, keep it human, keep it short and keep the emphasis on listening.

(Keith Nichols 2003: 91)

Introduction

In this chapter, we identify and explore some of the fundamental interpersonal skills under-pinning psychological caregiving: communication skills, assessment skills; emotional care skills; counselling skills; and informational care skills. We should make clear here that there are many excellent texts on the market that focus exclusively on communication and counselling skills in the caring professions. What follows is in no way a comprehensive coverage of these. Rather, it aims to highlight a range of skills that research has shown underpin effective psychological caregiving. Readers are directed to the reference list at the end of the book for texts providing more detailed coverage of communication and counselling skills. We begin by exploring the broad notion of 'interpersonal skills' as they might operate within health care contexts.

Interpersonal skills

Before we can describe 'interpersonal skills' it is perhaps helpful to consider exactly what we mean by a 'skill', as this might help us to distinguish between skills and personal qualities.

Reflection point

What are your skills? What makes them skills?

You may have identified skills such as playing a musical instrument, taking a blood pressure, driving a car, or playing a sport. Personal qualities, we have noted in the previous chapter, are to a large degree inborn (although they can be modified over time). Skills, on the other hand, are learned rather than innate; they can be developed through practice until competence is achieved, but there is not necessarily an end point; we can continue to improve on our performance.

These features also apply to interpersonal skills: they are skills that we learn and practise and which can constantly improve. However, unlike the skills of playing a musical instrument or riding a bike which can be undertaken alone, they always involve the 'connection between two or more people or groups and their involvement with one another' (Bach and Grant 2009). Nolan (2000) showed that being interpersonally skilled was fundamental to the caregiving role, and that being interpersonally competent in health care comprised skills such as 'getting to know you', 'establishing trust', 'anticipating need' and 'going the extra mile'.

While we might expect that anyone choosing to enter a health care profession probably already has good interpersonal skills and is 'interpersonally competent' in this way, this cannot be taken for granted. As we have noted in previous chapters, many complaints are received by the Parliamentary and Health Service Ombudsman about poor interpersonal skills on the part of health care professionals (http://www.ombudsman.org.uk/about-us/publications/annual-reports). We will consider some of the reasons for this in Chapter 9, but for now, let us try to unpick what we mean by interpersonal skills in the context of health care.

In Chapter 4 we explored Nichols' model of psychological caregiving and the findings of Priest's (2001) study, in which the central elements of assessment and monitoring, information giving, emotional care, and basic counselling were uncovered. Implicit within these aspects of care are some essential underpinning skills. For example, in order to be able to provide the right information to the right person in the right way at the right time, we need to have good communication skills. To be able to provide emotional care and to offer basic counselling, we need to have good observation skills and active listening skills. The effective practitioner will eventually be able to combine these skills in an almost unconscious way in the process of becoming an 'expert' caregiver (Benner 1984), having first learnt, practised, and then internalised each one. But for clarity, it is often helpful to consider each skill separately and in depth, and we begin by exploring communication skills.

Communication skills

In one sense, everything in this chapter could have been subsumed under the heading 'communication skills', but in this section we explore the skills that many people would instinctively think form part of communication: listening and talking to others. We consider also the skills of identifying and interpreting non-verbal communication – body language, facial expression, posture, gestures and personal presentation – that enable us to make as full an assessment of our patients' needs as possible.

Communication can be defined as 'a process that involves a meaningful exchange between at least two people to convey facts, needs, opinions, thoughts, feelings or other information through both verbal and non-verbal means, including face-to-face exchanges and the written word' (Department of Health 2010). It is the foundation of effective health care practice because health care is an interpersonal activity and very little of a carer's role does not involve at least one other person (try thinking of elements of your own role that do not!).

Action point

What is communication for? List as many functions as you can.

Broadly, communication can have any or all of the following functions:

- *Task completion* – Getting something done for our own benefit, such as asking for help in a shop or asking someone to babysit for us.
- *Control* – Getting someone else to do something for their benefit, such as changing an unhealthy behaviour.
- *Information exchange* – Giving and receiving information.
- *Expression of thoughts or feelings* – This enables us to get closer to others and to develop empathy with others' situation.
- *Reducing anxiety* – Often by expressing thoughts and feelings, we are able to feel that 'a problem shared is a problem halved'.
- *Social/pleasure* – While we may be content with our own company for some of the time, most experiences are enhanced if they are shared with others or discussed with others.
- *Ritual* – This function helps us to know the accepted ways of responding in given situations – so, for example, we know that when we meet someone for the first time we should say 'how are you' or 'pleased to meet you', or similar.

In most everyday communication, several functions co-exist in the same communication or 'message transfer'. For example, while we are giving someone driving directions, we may be reducing their anxiety about getting lost as well as providing factual information; while we are sharing our thoughts about a TV programme we have watched with a friend, we are at the same time experiencing social interaction and hopefully having a pleasurable experience! The same is largely true of professional communication, but for now we will focus on individual functions.

Action point

Reflecting on your caregiving experience, for each of the functions of communication listed above, identify *one* example of how you might communicate to achieve that function.

Some of these functions are easier to apply to practice than others. For example, most health care professionals would readily identify with the 'information exchange' function of communication, as it happens so frequently in most contexts: we ask patients to provide us with information about their personal circumstances and health problems, and we share with them information about what will happen to them during their health care experience.

Perhaps functions such as 'control' may seem somewhat unpalatable in the context of health care. However, we might use our communication skills to persuade someone to do something that is in their best interests, such as stopping smoking or adopting a more healthy diet. On occasion, we might use the 'control' function in an emergency situation, where we need to direct people to take action very quickly (such as shouting 'look out!' when something is about to fall on someone's head). Other functions, such as 'alleviation of anxiety' are highly relevant in health care settings where such emotions are often heightened.

Structure of human communication

All human communication needs certain elements to be in place: a message that is to be transmitted between two or more people; a sender of the message; a receiver of the message; and an appropriate transmission channel or form in which to send the message. The sender's role is first to encode the message in such a way that the receiver can 'hear' and understand it, and second to select the appropriate form or channel of communication. There also needs to be feedback from the receiver to the sender to indicate that the message has been understood, and an awareness of ways in which the environment or context can affect message transmission.

There is clearly potential for breakdown to occur at any stage of the process: for example, if we have not encoded the message correctly; if we have used the wrong form or channel of communication; if the receiver is unable to decode and therefore understand the message; if the receiver does not provide feedback to indicate they have received the message correctly; or if there are environmental constraints such as noise, pain, or anxiety. It would be inappropriate and ineffective, for example, to give a message in written form to someone who could not see, or read, or who was unconscious. Alternative forms of communication such as touch, however, would be an appropriate means of transmitting messages in all of these situations.

Forms of communication

Most of the examples in the list above, and perhaps your own examples, involve spoken or oral communication. You might also have considered the many occasions when health care professionals use the written word to communicate, such as in writing care plans, or producing health educational materials. Both oral and written communication can be subsumed under the heading 'verbal communication' because they involve words.

However, from the Department of Health (2010) definition above, it is clear that what we say in words forms only a part of the whole spectrum of communication. Many would say, in fact, that spoken words form only around 30 per cent of human communication (see, for example, Argyle 1988), and that the most prevalent and powerful form of communication is in fact 'non-verbal communication'.

Non-verbal communication (NVC) is used both to reinforce the spoken word and, in many cases, to replace it. Imagine, for example, that you have received bad news and are crying. There is unlikely to be, at that moment, anything that another person can say to change the situation or to make you feel better, but someone putting their arm round your shoulder or giving you a hug can communicate very powerfully that they are with you and offering you support. NVC can also be used to warn of impending action; if we observe someone pacing the room with their fists clenched and an angry facial expression, we may need to anticipate them becoming verbally or physically aggressive, and prepare to intervene to prevent this from happening if possible.

NVC can be expressed in a number of different ways, including:

- paralanguage (the *way* we express ourselves verbally – tone of voice; pitch; pace; speed);
- the way we use our body (kinesics), such as eye contact, facial expression, gestures and posture;
- the way we use the space between us and those with whom we are communicating (proxemics);
- the way we use (or do not use) touch;

- the way we present ourselves to the outside world, such as how we dress and the possessions we have around us.

Because NVC is a largely *unconscious* form of communication, it is more difficult to manage or hide from others than the spoken word. So, if there is a mismatch between the words someone uses and their non-verbal communication, the non-verbal communication is likely to covey the most accurate and reliable message. Unfortunately, most adults are thought to be insensitive to non-verbal cues (we may recognise them, but fail to interpret or respond to them), so it is especially important that health care professionals become skilled at identifying, interpreting, and responding to the non-verbal message, especially when it is at odds with what the person is saying.

As communication should always be a two-way process, where possible, we need to consider not only how our patients use the various forms of communication in their interactions with us, but also how we use our communication skills in our interactions with them. In sum, communication in all its forms underpins effective psychological care, and allows us to identify and respond appropriately to our patients' psychological needs. Understanding the structure, functions, forms, and process of effective human communication can help us to deliver effective psychological care. We now move on to explore ways in which, using these communication skills together with observation skills, psychological needs can be assessed.

Psychological assessment skills

Assessment, in relation to health care, is the collection of information about a patient's health status, which is then analysed and interpreted by the carer, allowing an initial judgment or formulation of holistic care needs to be made and a plan for addressing these needs to be drawn up. The accurate perception and recognition of a patient's needs, whether expressed overtly or not, has been identified as a central attribute of caring (Sadler 1997). To be able to recognise our patients' need for care, we should possess finely tuned observation skills and be able to incorporate these into our patient assessment strategies. Assessment is often considered to be one of the most important interactions a carer has with a patient because it sets the tone for all subsequent interactions, as well as providing baseline information from which to determine care needs.

In relation to psychological needs, the assessment process aims to 'determine the normal psychological functions that are being affected by current health status, with a view to identifying specific psychological needs' (Bach 1995). Hence, it is necessary to have at least a basic understanding of 'normal psychological function' in order to judge how these are being affected by ill health, and we consider this further in Chapter 7. Furthermore, Nichols (1993) believed that not only assessment, but also continuous monitoring of patients' psychological state is required in all nurse–patient encounters such that they are able to identify problems and decide upon the appropriate intervention or refer on to an appropriate agency or service.

Action point

What might you notice about a patient you were assessing that would indicate their psychological needs?

You may have identified some elements that would be obvious to a passing stranger: your patient's physical appearance, for example. Does he or she appear clean and well nourished? Or dishevelled, dirty, and in need of a shave? While such observations might relate directly to patients' physical health status, they can also be indicative of their psychological state – perhaps they feel low in mood or anxious, and taking care of their physical appearance is not high priority. The passing stranger may also be well able to observe aspects of the patient's behaviour; such as if they appear agitated or restless, unable to settle and pacing up and down.

Perhaps the passing stranger may not notice, though, less obvious features such as the patient's facial expression: are they smiling, frowning, grimacing as though in pain? Are they able to make and maintain eye contact? Are they showing interest in what is going on around them, or do they appear to be withdrawn or focused only on themselves? All of these elements can give a deeper insight into patients' emotions. When you enter into conversation with them, how does their mood seem? Do they seem to be low in mood, or flat? Does their mood seem to fit the situation they are in? Is their mood fluctuating between happy and sad? Can you read any particular emotions in their facial expressions, such as fear, anger, suspicion, or sadness? Other elements of psychological functioning that may be picked up during assessment could be described as cognitive: how well the patient can concentrate and attend to what we are saying and to what is going on around them; how well they are oriented to their surroundings; how much understanding and insight they appear to have about their situation and future; and how good their memory appears to be.

In picking up these signs and perhaps exploring further in your communication with your patient, you are effectively assessing (and subsequently monitoring) your patient's psychological state. The quotation from Nichols (2003), with which this chapter opened, suggests the key principles that underpin assessment of patients' psychological state: simple, human, short, with an emphasis on listening. Nichols suggests that the information we need to gather from our observations and assessment in this way concerns the patient's emotional state or mood; their outlook and expectations; any psychological difficulties they may be experiencing; and any action to be taken. Nichols (2003: 93) provides a sample data sheet on which to record the assessment. A simple care plan arising out of Priest's work (2001) is shown in Figure 6.1.

While we as health carers are not normally psychiatrists or psychologists and thus not expected to identify or diagnose mental health problems, it is helpful as a minimum to be able to assess accurately for the presence of anxiety and depression, since these are two common emotions in health care settings. A broad awareness of the common symptoms and presentations of anxiety and depression will be useful in all health care contexts. We will then be in a better position to pass our observations on and perhaps instigate a referral process.

Recognising depression

Depression is a disorder of mood or 'affect', and is the most commonly experienced 'affective disorder'. Some people experience episodes of *mania* or *hypomania*, where the mood is abnormally elevated. Depression and mania are thought to be contrasting manifestations of the same problem, and people who experience episodes of both depression and mania or hypomania are said to suffer from *bipolar disorder* (in the past, this was referred to as manic-depressive illness), while those who predominantly experience episodes of depression are said to suffer from *recurrent* or *unipolar depression*.

Depression is a mood state that is outside the range of normal mood, either in duration or severity, or both. It is important to be aware of the distinction between depression as a

1 Assessment of psychological need:	2 What might be the reason(s) for this?	3 How does this need usually show itself?	4 Psychological care intervention(s) to address this need:	5 Evaluation: how effective was the intervention?

a) *Emotional*
e.g. Is the patient
  – Anxious/frightened?
  – Sad/low/depressed?
  – Angry/feeling guilty?
  – Other
 	
b) *Cognitive*
e.g. Is the patient
  – Confused?
  – In need of information?
  – Other				

Figure 6.1 Psychological care plan

Column 2: Would include carer's tentative interpretations based on knowledge of the patient/family/background; observations and questioning, as appropriate.

Column 3: Would include observations such as crying; asking for reassurance; aggression; restlessness etc.

Column 4: Should include specific interventions such as giving time/attention, listening, counselling, giving information, liaising with family; acting as an advocate (in all cases detailing what/how much/how often/by whom/when to review), as well as referral to other agencies.

disorder or problem, and the normal mood changes and associated responses everyone experiences when they have bad news or experience a loss or change in their lives. We can all say that we 'feel depressed' when in fact what we are experiencing is ordinary and appropriate sadness or unhappiness. Even when there has been a major precipitating factor or loss, such as bereavement, the grief reactions and low mood that follow are normal and will usually resolve in time. It is this normal response that we are perhaps most likely to experience in our patients, as many will be dealing with one or a number of loss factors (including temporary loss of home, family, and normal routines, if they have been admitted to hospital).

Depression as a 'problem', though, is very common, so it is likely that at least some of our patients will be experiencing a form of depression that has moved outside the range of 'normal response to loss'. Based on UK statistics, depression occurs in 1 in 10 adults or 10 per cent of the population in Britain at any one time, with lifetime prevalence somewhere between 1 in 6 to 1 in 4 (MIND 2010). Women are twice as likely as men to experience depression, but the figures for depression in men are rising. Nonetheless, it is a treatable problem; the prognosis for someone with depression is good, even though the condition tends to be recurrent.

Depression and physical illness

Despite these figures, depression often goes unrecognised, both by the person experiencing it and by health care professionals. It may manifest itself as a physical problem, such as headache or fatigue, so individuals may not seek or receive appropriate help. Furthermore, some physical illnesses are especially associated with depression, such as multiple sclerosis, Parkinson's disease; hypothyroidism; and some disabling illnesses such as rheumatoid arthritis. Additionally, some prescription and illicit drugs can produce symptoms of depression. Knowing this will help us to be alert to the possibility in our patients.

Depression affects all areas of functioning: physical, psychological (emotional and cognitive), behavioural, and social.

Physical

Physical signs are often the first indication of problems, and include:

- fatigue and loss of energy;
- sleep changes (typically, there is a pattern of getting off to sleep reasonably well, but waking in the early hours and being unable to return to sleep);
- appetite and weight changes (usually, this is loss of appetite and consequent weight loss, but over-eating and consequent weight gain is not uncommon).

Clearly, many of these symptoms will be present in physical illness even when the person is not depressed, so it is important to consider our observations of such physical signs in conjunction with other evidence.

Emotional

Persistent low mood is the predominant symptom, although mood variation through the day is common in depression. It is often in the early morning when the person feels at their lowest, and this is often experienced in conjunction with early morning waking. Loss of interest and pleasure in the usual activities, a sense of anxiety and irritability are all also common emotional experiences.

Cognitive

People with depression may experience low self-esteem and hold broadly negative beliefs, such as 'I'm useless', or 'things will never improve'. Commonly, they will experience loss of concentration, guilt, hopelessness, and sometimes suicidal thoughts.

Behavioural and social

There may be a loss of interest in activities, such that the individual will withdraw from everyday social situations. Some people may experience reduced motor activity: a slowing down of movements, speech, and gestures. Alternatively, some people will appear agitated and find it difficult to settle.

Recognising anxiety

Around 5 per cent of adults experience generalised anxiety disorders. As with depression, anxiety is more common in women than in men (MIND 2010). There are several different manifestations of anxiety; including panic disorder, obsessive-compulsive disorder, and phobias, but for now we will consider the most common form, generalised anxiety disorder.

Anxiety is a normal, adaptive response to threat, change, stress, or confusion, such as will be experienced by most people when they become ill and in need of health care services. It is a psychological and physiological state that anticipates real or imagined threat, and prepares the body to confront and deal with it or avoid it (we discuss stress and the stress response further in Chapter 7). Most people will, from time to time, feel stressed and anxious and question whether they have the ability or resources to cope, but can normally do so when they are able to draw on existing coping strategies and support systems. When this sense of being unable to cope becomes overwhelming, the person's anxiety may have gone beyond a 'normal' response to stress.

Anxiety is characterised by a persistent and sometimes overwhelming feeling of apprehension and a range of physical and psychological symptoms. Physical symptoms include:

- headache;
- nausea;
- dry mouth;
- muscular tension;
- sweating;
- palpitations;
- dizziness;
- hyperventilation;
- sleep disturbance (typically, difficulty in getting off to sleep).

Emotional symptoms include sensitivity to noise and restlessness, while cognitive symptoms include experiencing a sense of dread or fearful anticipation, repetitive worrying thoughts, and poor concentration.

It is important to note that while generalised anxiety is very common, in fact mixed anxiety and depression is the most commonly experienced mental health problem amongst adults in the UK, with around 9 per cent of people experiencing this combination of symptoms (MIND 2010). So we need to be alert to the possibility that given their experiences of illness, diagnosis, treatment, prognosis, and the many loss experiences associated with illness, our patients are likely to experience depression, anxiety, or both.

Tools to guide the psychological assessment process

Should we wish to delve further into our patients' emotional and cognitive states (depending on the context and our specific role within the organisation), there is a wealth of assessment tools often readily available within hospital settings. To identify the presence of depression or anxiety, for example, these include the General Health Questionnaire (GHQ, Goldberg and Huxley 1980), and the Hospital Anxiety and Depression Scale (HADS, Zigmond and Snaith 1983). Such tools have 'cut off' points; scores above which indicate potential problem areas and can thus provide a rapid indication of need for further intervention or referral. Other specific tools are the Beck Depression Inventory (BDI) (Beck *et al*. 1961), the Hamilton Anxiety Assessment (Hamilton 1959); and (to assess cognitive functioning including memory and orientation), the Mini Mental State Examination (MMSE; Folstein and Folstein 1975). Some of these tools require training to administer and may not all be available in every setting, but if they are available or have been used it is helpful to be aware of patients' scores and how these change over time.

We must bear in mind, however, that no matter how structured or comprehensive our assessment, important clues to psychological needs can be missed, perhaps because of a lack of time, as nurses in Priest's study commented:

> If you're on a busy ward, a very busy ward, people could get overlooked with their psychological needs. You're just trying to concentrate on the main physical [things].

> Sometimes I might miss something completely – sometimes you don't pick anything up and there could be quite a problem but you don't get to the bottom of it.

Equally, perhaps in line with Nichols' notion of 'masked reactions', we fail to perceive accurately or to question further:

> Because she was a confident person, maybe we presumed that she was, and I don't think she actually was really. So maybe we did handle it wrong, maybe we had too much of a joke with her – had too much of a laugh with her – not took her seriously enough – It might have been better to handle her with more – kid gloves really.

In summary, accurate assessment of patients' appearance, behaviour, cognitive processes and emotional state is a key skill in psychological care delivery. Assessment is aided if we have good observation skills and a baseline understanding of commonly experienced emotional states such as anxiety and depression. There are tools with which to collect and record observations and information as it arises, such as a dedicated psychological care plan or rating scale. We move on now to look in more depth at the skills needed to identify patients' emotional state and to respond appropriately.

Emotional care skills

As we have noted, in the process of assessing and monitoring our patients' psychological needs we will be paying particular attention to their emotional state. We have touched on the changes of mood and emotion experienced with depression and anxiety, but as carers we need to have skills in identifying and responding to a whole range of emotions that may be triggered as a result of illness.

Action point

What do you understand by the word 'emotion'? List some 'everyday' emotions experienced by humans.

Emotions are sometimes described as 'feelings'; common emotions are sadness, happiness, anger and fear. You may have produced a much longer list than this, and in fact in the quest to 'pin down' human emotions, some researchers have identified literally hundreds of 'emotion words'. However, on close examination, many of these words are describing very similar if not the same emotion, and there is a view that the entire range of possible human emotions can be reduced to a maximum of seven major headings: sadness, anger, fear, surprise, disgust, contempt and enjoyment. There is general agreement that these core emotions can be observed in facial expressions, and that they are observable in young babies, leading us to believe they are innate. There is also some agreement that they are universal – in other words, they are consistent in people across different cultures (Ekman 2004). Some writers propose that just five categories (sadness, happiness, anger, fear and disgust) are sufficient to capture the fundamental human emotions (Bach and Grant 2009). Our initial task, in providing emotional care, is to identify the correct emotion or set of emotions that our patient is experiencing.

Emotions, however, do not 'stand alone'. As we have noted when we considered depression and anxiety, they come as a package with physiological responses, thoughts (cognitions), and behaviours. So, for example, if someone *feels* frightened about their impending medical test results, they may experience the physiological symptoms of nausea or dizziness. They may *think* they are going to receive bad news and that this will mean their future health is in jeopardy. In response, they may *behave* by avoiding going to see the doctor so as to avoid the unpleasant news.

The stages of emotional care

Our initial task in providing emotional care is to identify the correct emotion or set of emotions that our patient is experiencing. Having done that, we then need to identify the depth of that emotion as it is experienced by the patient at that particular time. Third, we need to find ways to help our patients to express what it is they are experiencing emotionally. Finally, we need to respond to the emotion. The following sections consider how these skills may be performed.

Identifying core emotions

Often, the most effective way of identifying emotions is to ask about them directly. Although something of a cliché and perhaps overused, the question 'how are you feeling?' will some-times lead to a clear verbal response. However, we should always be aware that many patients adopt the 'culture of masked reactions' (Nichols 2003) and so we should not assume that because a patient says 'I'm fine, thanks', that the patient does actually feel fine. Indeed, not all patients are able to communicate how they feel verbally, so we need to be skilled in identi-fying and interpreting non-verbal communication as outlined earlier in this chapter. A further way in which we can identify core emotions is to explore the thoughts, physical sensations and response behaviours that accompany them, and thus tap into emotions indirectly. So, for example, if a patient reports that she feels nauseous and sweaty (because we know these are symptoms of anxiety, see above), we might ask her if anything is worrying her and thus invite her to share her emotions with us.

Finally, we may have access to observational tools that will help us to identify emotions experienced by our patients when they cannot be expressed in words. The 'Observed Emotion Rating Scale' (Lawton *et al.* 1999), for example, uses line drawings of a range of facial expressions with accompanying descriptions, for comparison with observations patients who cannot communicate verbally.

Identifying the depth of emotion – the continuum of human emotional responses

The second task, having identified the core emotion, is to determine the strength or depth of that emotion.

Action point

Choose one of the following core emotions: anger, happiness, sadness or fear. Make a list of all the words you can think of that are associated with that word. (Tip: for examples of alternative emotion words, try using the thesaurus built into most computer word processing packages.) Then place the words in order according to how strong a representation of that emotion you believe the word to be.

There are no absolute right or wrong answers, as these are just 'words' and cannot accurately convey an emotional state. However, taking the emotion word 'fear' as an example, some words associated with it might be: apprehension, terror, anxiety, nervousness, worry, concern, and panic. If we try to place them in 'strength' order along a continuum ranging from weak to strong, we might arrive at something like: apprehension, nervousness, concern, worry, anxiety, fear, panic and terror. We might want to add a word to convey the lack of that emotion, so we might insert 'calm' at the beginning of the continuum. Taking 'sadness' as another example, we might identify and order words associated with sadness in the following way; gloom, unhappiness, sadness, depression, misery, wretchedness.

Action point

Try this exercise yourself with another emotion, such as anger or happiness.

As previously discussed, there are many rating scales available that attempt to objectify the depth of emotion experienced. The HADS (Zigmond and Snaith 1983), for example, aims to provide an objective measure of someone's level of both anxiety (the fear emotion) and depression (the sadness emotion); very useful when we are aware that mixed anxiety and depression is common. However it is relatively simple to ask the patient for a practical illustration, such that when they tell you they are anxious, you ask them to rate their anxiety on a scale from 0–10, with 0 being (for example) 'completely calm' to 10 being 'the worst anxiety you can imagine'. In this way, we can gain a better sense of their perception of the emotion and how it is experienced by them at the time, and furthermore, use this measure as a baseline with which to compare how they feel on subsequent occasions.

Facilitating emotional expression

A third component of emotional care is encouraging patients to express their emotions rather than keep them hidden, so that we can ensure that they feel listened to and understood. This will go some way towards helping them deal with unpleasant emotions that may exacerbate physical symptoms, increase pain and harm recovery. Bennett (1994: 478) suggested that emotional care involved 'providing an environment in which the patient is given permission to explore some of the negative emotions arising from their illness'. This would, in addition, promote a sense of safety and control.

However, there is a problem with the use of the word 'negative' in relation to the emotions experienced in illness, in that it suggests an undesirable state that must be corrected or reversed. In order to provide appropriate emotional care, we must accept that it is normal and usual for people to experience strong emotions when encountering stressful situations such as illness or loss, and that the expression of these emotions has an important therapeutic function (Nichols 1993). In the next section of this chapter, we explore fundamental components of counselling skills, such as active listening, paraphrasing and reflecting, that can help facilitate emotional expression.

Providing emotional support

The final stage of the emotional care package is to provide emotional support. This can be done effectively in an informal manner. Nichols (1993) suggested that emotional care did not call for much intervention. Its objective, not entirely passive, is to 'allow patients to express feelings in a safe, supportive atmosphere, in order that they are not isolated with their troubles and can make progress with the emotional tasks created by illness and injury' (Nichols 1993: 154). According to Nichols, the specific skills required of carers in providing emotional care include making the patient feel safe, giving permission for emotional expression, helping patients get in touch with their emotions, showing understanding and acceptance, and sharing personal feelings.

Emotional care can be provided more formally in some health care contexts. For example, Pålsson and Norberg (1995) examined the effects of a structured programme of emotional support for women newly diagnosed with breast cancer. Such emotional support comprised giving them the opportunity to talk about their illness, to express and identify feelings of anxiety and to understand the connection between symptoms and the illness. This opportunity was facilitated by nurses listening, consoling, answering questions and explaining misunderstandings, coupled with the identification of patients' personal resources and coping strategies. Nurses were specifically trained to carry out these interventions.

One of the most effective ways of providing emotional support is by communicating empathy, both verbally and non-verbally, in the ways we have outlined in Chapter 5 and will consider further in the next section.

Counselling skills

Our discussion of emotional care leads us directly into a consideration of the next set of skills outlined in this chapter – counselling skills. Counselling can achieve many things, such as helping patients to understand and accept that certain feelings are a 'normal' consequence of their illness or injury (Harrison 2001), but it is above all using listening and responding skills to encourage people to share their emotions about the situation they find themselves in. As one nurse commented: 'All nurses should be equipped with basic counselling skills to help them to relate and communicate with the patients on more than a superficial level'.

According to Burnard (2005), who has researched and written extensively about counselling in health care over the past 30 years, counselling is a process 'in which one person helps another to clarify his or her life situation and to decide further lines of action' (Burnard 2005: 2). So, counselling is a process, not a one-off activity, and one that requires a combination of skills, personal qualities and procedures. Let us think about the sorts of situations and problems that counselling skills might be used to help.

Action point

Make a list of as many human problems/concerns as you can. Think about your own life experiences as well as those you have encountered in your workplace.

Mark *Y* those for which you think it would be helpful to meet to talk about with another person to clarify the problem or concern and consider appropriate actions. Mark *N* those for which it would not. Count up the number of *Y*s and *N*s.

From this exercise, it is likely that you have identified more *Y*s than *N*s. You may have concluded that most issues/concerns can be usefully explored (*not* necessarily solved) in this way with another person, and that counselling may therefore be relevant in many if not all areas of human life and indeed health care. However, counselling perhaps has particular relevance in contexts where people have to face major changes or adjustments: life-threatening illnesses, disfiguring conditions, disabilities, and losses of various forms (such as loss of function, loss of future, loss of a partner or relative, or loss of potential). Clearly, in many of these situations, no amount of counselling can 'solve the problem'; rather, counselling is a vehicle for helping the person to explore their situation and the thoughts and feelings surrounding it, in an understanding atmosphere provided by the counsellor. Burnard (2005) makes the point that no one can be 'counselled' unwillingly; a fundamental pre-

requisite is that the individual must have a willingness to engage in the counselling relationship, and a desire to change in some way, even if this is only by coming to terms with a
difficult situation. Hence, counselling is a purposeful activity, but the purpose comes from
the client, not the counsellor.

We have said that counselling is a process, and there are many approaches to counselling
(psychodynamic, cognitive-behavioural, and humanistic, to name but a few – refer back to
Chapter 2 for more on these psychological approaches), and indeed many models of the
counselling process (e.g. Rogers, Egan, Carkhuff). The key elements, however, are likely to
be as in Figure 6.2. This might serve as an 'eclectic' model for counselling, and we will then
explore the discrete elements of the process in more detail.

Creating the environment

What do we mean by 'the environment' in a counselling context? To some extent, this refers
to the physical environment. In an ideal world, we would all have access to private,
confidential rooms with comfortable chairs, with tea and coffee on tap, where we could take
our patients when we recognise that they have a need to talk to us about their concerns. Such
an environment is typical of the counselling or therapy rooms provided in GP surgeries or
other health care establishments. However, few clinical areas in hospitals have access to such
dedicated spaces, even were all our patients physically well enough to leave their beds to get
to them, and even if we could offer such dedicated time to this sort of activity. So how can
we offer appropriate environments in which our patients will feel comfortable to open up to
us and not be concerned about lack of privacy? We have to be creative with the use of space,
compensate for the lack of facilities as much as we can, and above all create an appropriate
'emotional environment'. As we will see in Chapter 7, we are predisposed to make very rapid
and lasting initial judgments of others, based on very little information; the saying that 'first
impressions are lasting impressions' is relevant when our patients are forming their impressions of us. So in our initial overtures to our patients, we are setting the scene and providing
the emotional environment in which they will, or will not, feel able to open up to us in
expressing their concerns.

- Creating a helping relationship
  - Creating the environment
  - Communicating 'core conditions' (Congruence, Empathy, Unconditional Positive Regard'
    [UPR])
- Exploring the problem by
  - Attending
  - Listening (including paraphrasing, reflecting, clarifying, summarising)
- Achieving shared understanding
- Action
- Ending

Figure 6.2 The counselling process

Reflection point

Can you recall an occasion where you met someone for the first time and felt that you had not really 'hit it off' or 'got off on the wrong foot'? Can you identify what it was that made this initial encounter unsuccessful?

According to Kagan and Evans (1998) and Hargie (2010), our initial or opening encounters with others are highly structured episodes that contain ritualised behaviours (handshakes, for example), and are shared across many cultures (though clearly the handshake example is not always appropriate cross culturally). They have both task and social functions; that is, they serve to put people at their ease, and open up the potential for an ongoing relationship (the social function), but also facilitate future behaviour, such as obtaining the patient's permission to given an injection or record a blood pressure (the task function). As you may have reflected, though, it is very easy for opening encounters to go wrong – perhaps because we have failed to greet the person properly, or introduce ourselves by name and role, or explained our purpose for meeting with them, or taken steps to put them at their ease. We should remain alert to the fact that these crucial early moments can set the pattern for our subsequent interactions and relationship with our patients, and ultimately, influence their satisfaction with our care.

Communicating core conditions

We have already explored the core conditions for effective counselling in Chapter 5: namely *congruence*: by communicating this the helper tries to ensure that all forms of communication (spoken, non-verbal) are congruent with one another; *unconditional positive regard*: a genuine acceptance of and respect for another human being, simply because they are a human being, and not judging them for any behaviours, attitudes or opinions that we may find difficult or unacceptable; and *empathy*: the ability first to see the world from another person's position or frame of reference, 'as if' we were that other person, and second, to communicate that empathic understanding to the other person in the relationship.

Exploring the problem

Having created the environment and communicated the core conditions, the effective counsellor is now in a position to begin to explore the problem in order to arrive at a shared understanding. Specific skills used at this stage of the process are attending and listening.

Attending

There are essentially three foci for our attention when we are engaged in communication with another person. First, we can focus attention inwards on ourselves and become preoccupied or distracted by our own thoughts, feelings and preoccupations. Second, we can focus our attention outwards towards the other person, but become distracted by fantasy – what we imagine about the other person, rather than what they are actually communicating to us. Third, we can focus our attention directly towards the other person, without letting either of these potential distractions interfere. This 'giving undivided attention' is actually very difficult to achieve.

Action point

Try giving undivided attention yourself with a willing friend or colleague. Take it in turns to really focus on the other person, including how they look, and what they are wearing, without making judgments or interpretations. Spend a few minutes describing what you are seeing to the other person. Afterwards, tell each other how it felt to give someone your full attention, and what it felt like to receive it.

This was an unnatural exercise but demonstrates the difficulty of really focusing on another person. You may have felt 'under the spotlight' and perhaps embarrassed by such focus on you. Perhaps this is because it is such a rare experience, we are unused to it and confused by it. But the ability to focus attention out to the other person is a fundamental prerequisite for listening skills, and deserves to be taken seriously and practised.

We can practise and enhance our attending skills by using appropriate non-verbal communication. Egan (2001), for example, advocated the SOLER position, where the letters in the acronym indicate:

- **S**itting squarely (this does not necessarily mean directly face to face, which can be seen as confrontational), but sitting upright and able to present your face clearly to the other person.
- Maintaining an **O**pen posture – this means not having arms or legs crossed (which can indicate 'I'm not really interested in you and am closed to what you want to tell me').
- **L**eaning forward – slightly, towards the other person, without exaggeration. This effectively communicates empathy.
- Making **E**ye contact – this is a social skill and needs to be at an appropriate level (it is estimated that more than 20 seconds of direct eye contact with another person can be experienced as uncomfortable and even threatening).
- **R**elax – easier said than done when you are focusing on all the other elements of the SOLER position – but with practice you will develop your own version of the position that is comfortable to you and allows you to feel as relaxed as possible in the situation.

Listening

Listening is an attentive activity and a fundamental communication skill, but in counselling we do not simply listen to the words that another person says to us. We should try also to focus on paralanguage (the way the words are spoken – pitch, tone, rate); the non-verbal messages (we 'listen' for the emotions underpinning what is said); and silence (what is not said), because, as we have previously noted, these factors are powerful components of the communication process. Effective listening should be active, that is, the listener tries not just to hear but also to assimilate and interpret what is transmitted through verbal and non-verbal channels. When we are listening, we should avoid being selective and listening only to what is of most interest to us, and should avoid 'pseudo listening', where we perhaps try to convey that we are listening with appropriate facial expression and body language, but are really focused in on our own thoughts and interests. This again is a difficult challenge. A further challenge is in allowing silence and not stepping in to fill it with our own commentary. Silence can be therapeutic, allowing both the one being listened to and the listener to collect their thoughts, reflect and consider where to go next. But silence should not be allowed to go on too long; judging the limits of helpful silence is in itself an important skill.

Skills of active listening

As well as communication, our availability and willingness to attend and listen, there are a number of techniques than can enhance listening, help the patient to feel 'listened to', and encourage them to continue to share their thoughts and feelings with us. These include:

- *Using minimal prompts*: this can be done verbally by saying things such as 'go on . . . ' or 'and then? . . . ' but it can also be done effectively with non-verbal means of communication such as nodding, leaning forward, and smiling.
- *Paraphrasing*: this is a technique of picking up and repeating elements of what the patient has said (their words rather than your interpretation of the words), in your own words. It demonstrates that you are listening and empathising. Sometimes it as simple as repeating the last few words that the patient has said, which often has the effect of encouraging them to continue their story. It might also be listening to longer elements of what they are saying, *summarising* in your own words, and presenting back to them with phrases such as 'what I'm hearing is . . .'; or 'so what you're saying is . . .'
- *Reflecting*: this is similar to paraphrasing but goes beyond the patients' words to your interpretation of the words and the emotional expression that may be behind them. It is a way of demonstrating listening to the feelings expressed and reflecting them back so that they can be *clarified.* For example, 'I get the sense that you are feeling [appropriate emotion word] . . . about what has happened'. Remember, though, from our discussion of emotional care, that it is not enough to identify the correct emotion; it is also necessary to judge the strength or depth of that emotion, so further reflection will aid this process. As an example, suppose we are listening to a patient's story about not being visited in hospital by a family member. You might say: 'It sounds as though you are feeling quite upset about this'. The patient then has the opportunity to confirm the emotion, or present an alternative, and indicate the strength of the emotion – for example, 'I'm not just upset, I'm really angry about it'.

The therapeutic effects of simply listening cannot be overstated. How often have you been thanked by a patient and you have really had to stop and think, 'but what did I do?' You may have 'simply' provided time and attention, and really listened, a luxury in many people's busy lives (you might like to reflect upon the last time you felt really listened to). By this stage, if we have been able to give adequate time and attention in an appropriate atmosphere and environment, we should have gone some way towards exploring the problem and achieving shared understanding, and that in itself can be therapeutic and indicative of good psychological care. We may be able to go further and explore future options with the patient, but we may here be going beyond the use of 'counselling skills' and into 'counselling' in its own right – something that few professional carers have the expertise, training or time to engage with in busy health care settings.

Can we all be counsellors?

An important distinction needs to be made between formal counselling, as practised by professional counsellors and therapists, and the use of counselling skills to facilitate effective communication, which can be practised by all nurses. The use of counselling skills with physically ill people is thought to have wide-ranging positive consequences, the benefits of which cannot be over-estimated (Bennett 1994, Watson 1994). However, there is much debate as to whether counselling skills should be acquired and practised by all nurses, or whether these are higher level communication skills needed only by some nurses. Nichols (1993) believed that all competent health care professionals should be equipped with basic counselling skills. Davis and Fallowfield (1991) similarly argued that counselling training was beneficial for improved communication by all health care professionals, a view shared by Morrison and Burnard (1997a), who agreed that all nurses needed counselling skills if they wished to be good communicators.

What counselling is not

A further distinction needs to be made between different uses of the term counselling. There is a view that counselling is essentially a directive approach involving the passing on of information or the giving of advice. This is in contrast to counselling as a non-directive, client-centred approach as advocated by Rogers and others, and outlined above. In this sense, counselling does not involve solving patients' problems, taking over responsibility for them, or giving false reassurance. It may be, though, that nurses have been trained and socialised into a 'doing' role whereby they are frustrated if they cannot solve patients' problems. Indeed, evidence from a small-scale study exploring nurses' attitudes to counselling suggested that some nurses were uncomfortable with a client-centred, facilitative interpersonal style, preferring instead a more prescriptive role (Morrison and Burnard 1997a). Nurses may, though, have doubts about their skills in this area and worry about saying the wrong thing. Nichols (1993) however, suggested that this was unlikely to happen, and that the practice of basic counselling techniques was well within the scope of most nurses.

Informational care

Patients recognise the need for information, and when invited to do so, readily complain about its lack. As we have previously noted, the Parliamentary and Health Service Ombudsman investigates concerns and complaints about the health service in England and reports that many concerns are about poor communication and information sharing. This will exacerbate the fact that people who are ill and anxious are already likely to process information in an atypical manner, so that their usual strategies for listening and remembering are altered (Gardner 1992). The positive effects of adequate information-giving are well documented, and include promoting recovery, reducing the severity of physical symptoms, anxiety and depression, reducing the length of hospital stay; reducing stress and over-pessimistic expectations; and even preventing illness (e.g. Bennett 1994, Boore 1978, Hayward 1975, Hyland and Donaldson 1989, Morris, Goddard and Roger 1989 Wilson-Barnett 1981). It has, thus, long been recognised that keeping a patient fully informed will, in conjunction with good physical care, help to ensure that care needs are met. Devine's (1992) meta-analysis of 191 studies, referred to in Chapter 4, exploring the effects of psycho-educational care for surgical patients (defined as the provision of health care information, skills teaching and psycho-social support) confirmed that there were significant benefits associated with the provision of such information and support in terms of speed of recovery, reduction of pain, reduction of psychological distress and reduction in the length of hospital stay.

However, before accepting without question that information giving per se is an essential component of psychological care, we must be aware that people differ widely in their information preferences and needs. It is common to find explicit guidance that '*all* patients *must* be told about their operation whether they like it or not (Hallett 1991), without adequate consideration of what, how much, when or how that information should be given. It is necessary, therefore, to consider the interaction between the amount, content and timing of information provided and individual patients' needs. These needs might be related to their coping style or 'locus of control' (Rotter 1966). In this theory, people with an internal locus of control believe that they can control events, while people with an external locus of control, conversely, believe that events are outside of their personal control.

For example, a patient with an internal locus of control who needs a surgical procedure might need specific, detailed information well in advance of the procedure, so that they know what to expect, and can perhaps do some of their own research on the internet or by asking others, and thus stay as much prepared for and in control of events as possible. On the other hand, a patient with an external locus of control may prefer to receive relatively simple information and reassurance nearer the time, so as to avoid potentially unpleasant information that they feel they have no control over until the last minute (Mitchell 2005). Likewise, studies have shown that 'monitors' (people who actively seek information) and 'blunters' (people who avoid information) need different amounts and types of information prior to procedures (Davis, Maguire, Haraphongse and Schaumberger 1994). These styles can be assessed using tools such as that developed by Miller (1987). Furthermore, in the context of the contemporary 'patient choice' agenda (NHS 2010), patients should be offered a choice regarding the package of information required, taking into account what is happening or will happen, what the patient is likely to experience, and what to expect in the future (Mitchell 2005).

We need, therefore, to consider on an individual basis:

- **what** information we give (content)
- **who** we are giving it to
- the **type** of information (structure, format, media)
- **how much** information to give
- **when** to give the information (timing)
- **how often** to give the information (frequency)
- **confidentiality issues** (who else needs to know/can know)

(Priest 2010)

While the precise details will vary for each situation, some general principles apply to them all. These include:

- Preparing the physical environment (privacy, comfort, time)
- Identifying the patient's beliefs and understandings
- Discovering patients' prior experience and expectations
- Giving specific rather than general information
- Stressing important content and repeating it as required
- Giving important information first and repeating it last

- Checking the appropriateness of language
- Providing back up material (written information, pictures, diagrams, demonstrations) for later reference
- Providing opportunity for questions

(adapted from Ley 1988 and Priest 2010)

Action point

Think of a patient you recently cared for. Using these principles, describe in writing the specific information this patient needed, and how you delivered that information. Would you do anything differently?

We should remember that giving information is only part of the story. As we have learned from the basic model of communication, there needs to be evidence that our information has been received and interpreted correctly, and therefore understood. In illness, patients' ability to receive information can be affected by any or all of their personality, their emotional state, their coping style and skills; their beliefs about health and illness; their cognitive ability (such as intelligence level or memory); the nature of their specific illness (sensory impairments and pain can get in the way); and any external features of the care setting (such as noise or overheating). Thus we need to be aware of these constraints and be patient when we need to repeat information or present it in a different way. In summary, as demonstrated by experienced nurses below, information giving and achieving understanding is an essential component of care.

> It's their need to know, be fully aware of all the information they can get. So they need to have an awareness of why they're in our ward, anyway, in hospital. Instead of just being shunted about we like them to be able to say why they're in hospital, to feel quite at ease with asking questions about why they're in there, and to . . . be fully aware, really.

> I think we should talk to them, explain everything that's going to go on or may possibly go on, that's the key to communication. Every nurse should do that routinely as part of the job. Just by talking and keeping everybody informed. That automatically, I've found out from experience, reduces the stress, well what's going on with me, I want to know, I want to know.

Summary

In this chapter, we have explored some of the interpersonal skills that are necessary for carers to possess in order to assess psychological needs and deliver effective psychological care. We have noted that in many cases these skills are demonstrated in combination, and there is clear overlap between them – for example, when does emotional care become counselling? Equally, there is overlap between what we might consider to be personal qualities (as discussed in Chapter 5) and interpersonal skills. In the next chapter, we complete the triad of 'qualities, skills, and knowledge' for psychological caregiving by considering what specific knowledge might help us to become effective psychological caregivers.

7 Knowledge for psychological care

All the ''ologies' in nurse education ignore much of what nurses and patients know makes a difference.

(Biley 2005: 17)

Introduction

Is the statement from Biley (above) true? Is there a place for ''ologies' (or in other words, scientific knowledge) in patient care? In Chapters 5 and 6 we explored the personal qualities and interpersonal skills that are necessary for effective psychological caregiving. We now turn, in this chapter, to explore the underpinning knowledge that health care professionals and students might need to draw upon in order to support and enhance these personal qualities and skills, and in turn, to contribute towards their psychological care delivery activities. In keeping with the focus of this book, the knowledge base of psych*ology* (rather than any other ''ology') will provide the illustrative material, but it is fully acknowledged that many other academic disciplines contribute to effective holistic care delivery. Specifically, in this chapter, we investigate the psychological knowledge that can support psychological assessment and monitoring; emotional care; informational care; and relationship-based care.

Psychological knowledge in caring

Over the years, a number of views have been expressed about what knowledge health care professionals need in order to be competent and effective deliverers of psychological care. Wells (1983), for example, claimed that nurses needed to know a comparatively large number and variety of psychological facts and be able to relate them to nursing situations, and that this was needed in order for nurses to be able to assess psychological needs and solve problems accordingly. Wilson-Barnett (1983: 335) too, considered that 'psychological care is a poorly understood and managed aspect of nursing . . . nurses should be exploring and exploiting psychology to improve care'; they thus require an accurate appraisal of psychological knowledge and the skills to apply principles to individual patients. Webster (1991) believed that psychological knowledge would add to the body of nursing knowledge, and, in addition to enhancing the quality of nursing practice, would also positively influence research, management and education. However, what seems to be missing is detail about what type of psychological knowledge is most relevant, how it should be taught, and how its application in practice should be facilitated in order to have an impact upon care. Many books provide a comprehensive introduction to psychological knowledge, both in its pure form and as applied to the caring professions. This chapter makes no attempt to be comprehensive, but takes instead a selective approach to psychological knowledge by focusing upon the areas that might best support the pre-requisite qualities and skills that we have identified as central to psychological care in Chapters 5 and 6.

Knowledge for assessment and monitoring

To be able to assess another person's needs, we need to have an understanding of the nature of both social perception and attitudes. Social perception can be defined as the way in which humans think about other people and make sense of their actions in a social context (Gross and Kinnison 2007), while attitudes can be defined as the evaluations we make about objects (including people) in our social world. Both of these mechanisms have a part to play in 'sense-making': how we explain other people's behaviours to ourselves and how we respond on the basis of these explanations. We will first explore social (or interpersonal) perception.

Social perception

Action point

Pick up a recent newspaper or magazine and select at random a photograph of a person that you don't know (avoid well known people such as celebrities, and try to avoid reading any of the headlines or text associated with the photograph).

   Jot down on paper your ideas about:

This person's name.

Their job.

The type of home they live in.

Whether you would like them if you met them at a social event.

Most people find this sort of exercise relatively easy, and it is perhaps worrying that we can so readily decide whether we would like someone or not from a one-dimensional image on paper and no other information. We are also very ready to ascribe social status (deciding, for example, that someone probably lives in a high rise council flat rather than a mansion, or works as a postman rather than a financial executive, based simply on appearance).

   Evidence suggests that when we first meet someone new, we make a quick assessment of what that person is like, drawing on very little information, and that we are subsequently quite reluctant to be proved wrong, even in the light of new information. Such a judgement is based on our own *implicit personality theory*, our understanding of people and how they behave. We may use quite superficial information on which to base our judgements, such as the clothes people are wearing, their address, and even their name (consider the difference, for example, between the names 'Tarquin' or 'Tallulah' and 'Terry' or 'Tracy'). Though most health care professionals would subscribe to a non-judgemental view of their patients, there are in fact many studies suggesting that people are treated differently within health care contexts according to how they look, how they behave, their age, social class and other such factors (Gross and Kinnison 2007).

Additionally, there are certain characteristics that appear to be most influential in making our judgement. In a famous study, Asch (1946) called these characteristics 'central traits' and they include qualities such as 'warmth' and its opposite, 'coldness'. Furthermore, if we perceive that someone possesses a positive central trait such as warmth, then we are also quite likely to assume they have other positive traits such as friendliness and kindness. If we perceive someone to have a negative central trait, such as 'coldness', we may also assume that they are unfriendly and unkind. This tendency is known as the 'halo effect'; we like to see people in as consistent a way as possible, so we make assumptions based on limited information. We need to bear in mind when meeting our patients and beginning the assessment process that first impressions are often inaccurate but are relatively enduring.

Stereotypes

As well as drawing on implicit personality theory to make judgements of individuals, we also draw on this theory as it applies to groups of people. A stereotype is a rigid and often negative generalisation about a group of people, and we use stereotypes as a quick way of classifying people, rather than having to make individual judgements about each new person we meet. Thus we tend to ignore individual differences in favour of assuming that characteristics are typical of all members of a particular group. Stereotypes are sometimes extreme caricatures of a group, with little relationship to reality. So for example, the stereotype of an 'Englishman' might be someone wearing a dark suit and a bowler hat, carrying a copy of *The Times* newspaper, while a 'Frenchman' may be someone wearing a beret and riding a bicycle, with a string of onions round his neck and a baguette in his hand.

Action point

Jot down a few notes on what a 'typical' nurse is like.

Nurses are generally thought of as female, and there are powerful and pervasive stereotypes portrayed in the media and popular culture, such as 'the battle axe', 'the ministering angel', 'the naughty nurse' and the 'doctor's handmaiden' (Bridges 1990). While such caricatures are mostly false, often humorous and perhaps harmless, the power of the stereotype is strong and can lead to more serious judgements being made based on an individual's membership of a particular ethnic or other identity group.

What is of more concern is how stereotypes can affect behaviour. Making a negative judgement of someone based on a group stereotype is only one step away from treating that person in a different and less favourable way than others; in other words, practising discrimination. This is contrary to the qualities and behaviours needed to provide effective psychological care, such as empathy, a non-judgemental approach, and unconditional positive regard (see Chapter 5). If we do treat someone in a less favourable way because of our stereotyped views, then this can in turn lead the person to behave in the way that we expect them to behave – an example of the self-fulfilling prophesy. Felicity Stockwell's (1984) landmark nursing research in the 1960s into why some patients were perceived as 'difficult' showed that it was *categories* of patients that were unpopular, so when a patient was judged to be a member of that category, they were deemed unpopular (and often treated differently) with little regard for their individual characteristics. Such categories of people were those with 'defects' such as deafness or mental health problems, those who had been in hospital for more than three months, and those who were 'foreign'. Jeffery (1979), too, in his shockingly titled paper 'Normal Rubbish', showed that patients who did not conform to expected patterns of 'normal sickness' and the legitimate sick role (for example, the 'over-doses'), were evaluated in a negative and sometimes hostile way by nurses in accident and emergency departments. Kelly and May's (1982) review of related literature identified groups of patients classed as 'bad': these included those who were incontinent, long-term sick, over dependent, or non-compliant. While such work has been criticised for ignoring the social context and the way in which we socially construct such labels (Johnson and Webb 1995), nonetheless it is important to be reminded of the ease with which we can make negative evaluations of individuals based on group characteristics, and the possible consequences in terms of poor quality care delivery.

Values, beliefs and attitudes

Values are our notions of what we believe to be good and desirable, and we will normally aim to act in accordance with our values. We are likely to hold just a few salient core values. So, for example, we might hold the value that 'it is wrong to physically hurt people', and we will try to act in accordance with this value by not deliberately hurting others. We might hold the value of 'honesty'; we will thus try to see ourselves as honest and try to be honest in our communications with others. Examples of nursing values might be:

- All patients are treated equally regardless of age, gender, race, illness, or disability.
- All patients should be treated the way we would wish to be treated ourselves.
- Nursing values the whole person.

You can probably think of others relating to this or your own profession.

Beliefs are the knowledge that we have about the world, such as that the world is round. We are likely to hold many beliefs. Of course, our beliefs are not always accurate, and generally change over time as new knowledge becomes available (for example, at one time, believing the word was flat would have been in accordance with current knowledge and therefore a reasonable viewpoint).

A major influence on the way in which we perceive and respond to people is our attitudes. Attitudes are our predisposition to see the world (and the people in it) in a particular way, based on our values and beliefs. Attitudes are always evaluative – it is not possible to have a neutral attitude towards someone or something. Hence we are predisposed to see people in a broadly positive or negative light, in accordance with our knowledge, experience, beliefs, values and expectations.

Attitudes are acquired through a variety of processes, including social learning (that is, observing and imitating the attitudes of others such as parents, teachers, peers, and people in the mass media); operant conditioning (we continue to hold attitudes that are reinforced); and social comparison (we tend to compare ourselves with others in order to judge whether our views are 'correct'). They serve many purposes, including providing us with predictability in the way we see the world and in allowing us to identify with others whose attitudes we share.

Attitudes are often thought to have three components – an affective (emotional) component; a cognitive (thinking) component, and a behavioural component. However, attitudes are not always good predictors of behaviour; people do not always do what their expressed attitudes might lead you to expect they will do. For example, a nurse might express a negative attitude towards smoking, believing it to be detrimental to health, but he or she smokes. Therefore although people might have a predisposition to behave in a particular way, we cannot predict behaviour reliably from expressed attitudes. Perhaps this explains how a caregiver can tell colleagues of his or her dislike for a particular patient, but can deliver perfectly good care to that patient nonetheless.

Prejudice

Prejudice (literally meaning to 'pre-judge') is an extreme form of attitude, and one that is usually negative and hostile. Our prejudices are normally based on faulty generalisations or stereotypes and can lead to avoidance, discriminatory behaviours and ultimately attack or abuse. An example of the recipients of prejudice are people from races different from our own (racism); however there are countless other '-isms' prevalent in health care and beyond, such as ageism and sexism.

Action point

Do we all have prejudices? Think about any you may have and how they affect your interactions with patients.

As an example, you may have a prejudice against people who are obese, particularly if this gets in the way of their health and recovery from illness. If you are really honest, have you ever treated such people differently on account of their size and weight? Complained to colleagues because they are difficult to help mobilise? Or been irritated by their reluctance to make healthy choices from the daily menu? We may think of ourselves as essentially congruent and non-judgemental in our caring, but it is important to reflect on and monitor our own attitudes, prejudices and behaviours as we strive to be effective psychological caregivers. We should also remind ourselves that our attitudes and prejudice can often show, through 'non-verbal leakage': through our facial expressions, through the distances we create between ourselves and our patients, and our use (or non-use) of touch, for example.

We are all human, and just because we are in caring roles this does not mean that we are immune from making negative evaluations of people based on our implicit personality theory, stereotypes, attitudes and prejudices. So how do we reduce the negative effects of these, and prevent them from impacting adversely on our care delivery? It is a difficult task, but it is sometimes helpful to try to separate the person from the behaviour. This is what Carl Rogers was striving for in his desire to convey unconditional positive regard. We do not have to like or agree with everything that our patients do, but at their heart is a humanity that we can seek out, respect and respond to. We can also try to tap into the patient's experience and underlying universal emotions (through developing our empathic understanding, see Chapters 5 and 6), rather than focusing on the behaviour that we find unpalatable or unacceptable. For example, we might ask ourselves why patients who are obese find it difficult to lose weight. Is this because they have a low self image or are feeling sad or depressed? Do they feel that no one cares about them enough to bother what they look like or whether they are harming their health? Sometimes looking deeper than the behaviour and thinking about our own emotions and experience can help us to see beyond the behaviour to the person within.

Having explored some of the psychological principles that underpin and might affect the way we observe and assess our patients, we now turn to explore psychological knowledge of relevance to emotional care.

Knowledge for emotional care

To be able to identify emotions, facilitate emotional expression, and to give appropriate emotional care, it is helpful to have a fundamental understanding of the mechanism of human emotion. In this section we consider theories around emotion and as an example, explore the knowledge base around an emotional state – stress – an experience common to us all (and often experienced by people in the health care system, patients, relatives and staff alike).

Reflection point

What do we think of when we say people are 'emotional'?

We might think about the way people respond to an event – crying because they have received bad news, for example. Or we may think of people as being inherently 'emotional' – the sorts of people who react in quite a dramatic way to events around them. Sometimes we might call these people 'highly strung'; while not a very technical term, it is one that conjures up an image of someone who is never very far from tears or anger, for example.

We have already noted in Chapter 6 that emotions have a number of components: the subjective feeling, the cognitive (thinking) processes associated with the feelings, the associated physiological changes, and the outward manifestation (such as facial expression) or behaviour. Opinion has changed over the years in the light of extensive research as to which component comes first. The nineteenth-century James–Lange theory, for example, suggested that emotions are triggered by an external stimulus, which leads to physiological changes experienced as bodily sensations (heart racing, dry mouth, difficulty in breathing, for example). Our experience of these bodily changes then leads us to experience the emotion. In other words, 'because my heart is racing, I must be frightened'; or 'because I am crying, I must feel sad'.

To put this explanation to the test, imagine a situation where a tiger bursts through your door (the external stimulus). You experience all the physiological signs of fear that are produced by the sympathetic nervous system and by the release of the hormones adrenaline, noradrenaline and cortisol from the adrenal glands. A 'fight or flight' reaction is triggered and you experience the emotion of fear; and either tackle the tiger (unlikely) or try to escape from it, perhaps by leaping out of the window. Once the immediate danger is over, the body will return to its normal homeostatic state.

More recently, however, theories have suggested that our experience of emotion is more complex, and depends in part on how we interpret that experience (a process known as cognitive appraisal). In this process, we first identify that an experience or situation is emotionally arousing, and we then appraise both the meaning of it (will this tiger really eat me?) and whether we have the resources to cope (is there an escape route other than the door? Am I fit enough to climb out of that window?). We then reappraise the situation in the light of our answers to these questions and act accordingly.

Stress as a human emotional experience

As an example of a common emotional experience, we will examine stress, as this is something likely to be experienced by everyone within a health care context, including carers.

Action point

Think about a recent experience you have had that you considered to be stressful. Make a note of:

The event or experience itself

Your response to it (how did you feel, what did you think, what did you do?)

In undertaking this exercise, you have considered stress both as a stimulus and as a response, and we will consider both of these approaches in the next section, together with a consideration of the interaction between the two.

Stress as a stimulus

We experience stress when we perceive that there is an imbalance between the demands being placed upon us (the stimulus or stimuli; sometimes known as stressors) and the resources we feel we have to deal with them. As humans we have a huge capacity to cope with multiple stressful events and experiences as long as we have adequate coping mechanisms to deal with them, perhaps the most powerful and protective of which is emotional support from other human beings. We have previously noted that it is often 'the last straw that breaks the camel's back' – perhaps a small additional demand that exceeds the resources we have available to deal with it on top of everything else that needs to be dealt with. This applies even when the stressor is essentially positive – such as playing sport in a competition, or performing music in public. Indeed, there is a theory (Yerkes and Dodson 1908) that we need to have this sort of stress experience in order to give us a competitive edge or get the best out of our performance, and only when the stress is too great, or is one stress factor too many, will our performance be adversely affected. Furthermore, when we experience events over which we feel we have little or no control, or events that are unpredictable, our chances of experiencing stress are increased.

So what sorts of things can be considered as stressors? Stressors can be any event external to us; in the 1960s, Holmes and Rahé (1967) were interested in the link between the events people experienced that required some change to their lives, and the onset of illness. They drew up a list of 43 life events and tried to establish how much these events required readjustment if they were experienced within a given period (such as 6 or 12 months). Some of these events could be considered as positive – such as holidays or Christmas – but they all require adaptive behaviour or readjustment from the existing steady state. As a result of extensive testing within different populations, they produced the *Social Readjustment Rating Scale* (an online version is available for self completion at http://www.mindtools.com/pages/article/newTCS_82.htm). They concluded that a high score (300+) was associated with an 80 per cent increased risk of illness, injury or psychological disorder; while a score of 200–299 suggested an increased risk of 50 per cent.

How relevant is such research today? The use of this type of 'tick box' approach has been criticised in that it is often difficult to separate external events from other illness related factors such as diet, smoking, or genetic predisposition to illness. But it does remind us that factors that are a result of being ill and perhaps being in hospital, such as changing eating or sleeping habits, are in themselves stressors and can add to other illness-related worries and fears in creating a stress experience.

As well as external or environmental factors being potential stressors, there may also be characteristics of the individual that predispose them to stress. For example, Friedman and Rosenman (1974) set out to discover whether there was a stress prone personality and whether this had any relationship with illness. They were able to distinguish between the Type A personality – the 'high achiever', and the Type B personality – 'the dreamer'. Later research has identified a Type C ('the coper'; someone who has difficulty expressing emotions, particularly negative ones) and a Type T ('the thrill seeker') personality. The characteristics of someone with a Type A personality (now more often referred to as a Type A Behaviour Pattern (TABP; Gross and Kinnison 2007) include competitiveness, aggressiveness, and a sense of time urgency. Significantly, Friedman and Rosenman claimed to have discovered a link between the Type A personality and an increased likelihood of heart disease, though the relationship is not universally accepted nor fully understood. Other researchers (e.g. Temoshok 1987) claim to have identified links between, for example, Type C behaviour patterns and a tendency to develop cancer. While we are unlikely to be able to measure the personality characteristics or behaviour patterns of our patients in such depth, nonetheless as part of our assessment we may be able to make a judgement about how well and in what way they are expressing their emotions and to be alert if these seem under- or over-expressed. We can certainly, as part of our assessment, discover whether there are external stressors in the patient's life (in addition to the illness experience) and determine in what ways, and how effectively, the patient is coping with these stressors. Consider, for example, the older patient admitted to hospital whose major concern is who will be feeding her budgerigar while she is away from home. This worry may be more acute than the reasons for admission, and careful assessment can reveal such important information.

Stress as a response

As we have noted, stress affects us physically, psychologically (both emotionally and cognitively) and socially. Physically, it can affect any or all of our bodily systems and can lead to an increased risk of physical problems ranging from headaches and skin disorders to more serious conditions such as coronary heart disease. The relationship between stress and the immune system is well known, though not fully understood, and is associated with a whole range of illnesses from minor viral infections to cancer. Selyé (1956) was one of the first people to explain the body's response to stress in his General Adaptation Syndrome (GAS) theory, defined as 'the non-specific, stereotypical response of the body to any demand which is interpreted as a threat to physical or emotional homeostasis'. According to GAS, the body passes through a number of stages in response to threat:

- *Alarm Stage* – in which the body perceives the threat and changes itself into a defensive mode preparing for a fight/flight response triggered by the sympathetic nervous system and adrenal hormones. For example, the heart rate, breathing, and muscle tension increase, and sugar and fat are released to provide the body with the energy needed to act.
- *Resistance Stage* – in which the body attempts to restore its equilibrium. Once the initial threat has disappeared, the body relaxes slightly but remains mobilised so that its capacity to resist and adapt are still present.
- *Exhaustion Stage* – this stage occurs if the threat returns repeatedly, causing the alarm reaction to be elicited too intensely or too frequently over an extended period. Wear and tear will begin to set in and the body's ability to resist effectively will result in diminished immune and organ functions (depending on the individual's physical makeup and ability to cope). Ultimately, exhaustion, collapse and eventually death will occur, but at the very least, outcomes of GAS are a lowered resistance to illness, a tendency to feel tired and weak, long-term irritability and a pessimistic outlook.

Psychologically, stress can affect both emotional and cognitive functioning. For example, we may become forgetful, or unable to concentrate or pay attention to detail in our activities. We may be irritable, and experience low self-esteem, helplessness, and emotional exhaustion. It is likely that burnout, experienced by many health care professionals (a combination of emotional exhaustion, depersonalisation, and a reduced sense of personal accomplishment, Gross and Kinnison 2007) occurs as a result of long-term stress, reducing resilience and causing people to feel powerless in their working situation, which in turn exaggerates stress.

Having considered stress both as a stimulus and as a response, we now examine the interaction between the two.

Stress as an interaction between stimulus and response

The way in which stress stimuli and individual responses interact is very much based on an individual's appraisal of the stimulus and their ability to cope with it. What one person sees as a stress factor, another will not. Equally, what may not be seen as a stressor on most occasions may become a stressor if it is one of too many things to cope with. A number of theories help to explain this individual interaction.

Bandura's (1989) *Self Efficacy Theory*: This is the extent to which we feel able to act effectively and exercise control over life events. The theory suggests that we reflect on and interpret actions we have taken in the past to deal with stressful situations, and that this will determine how we behave and interact. If we feel we have been successful in the past, we are likely to believe that we can cope when similar situations arise in the present or future.

Seligman's (1975) *Theory of Learned Helplessness*: In his now controversial experiments, Seligman showed that dogs would become helpless if given repeated electric shocks from which there was no escape. They simply gave up trying, almost as though they thought 'what's the point; I've tried this before and it didn't work'. In relation to humans, it is thought that people who believe that they do not have control over life events are more vulnerable to the harmful events of life changes (Gross and Kinnison 2007). Seligman drew a connection between learned helplessness and depression in humans.

Rotter's (1966) *Locus of Control Theory*: Also relevant in terms of the way we interpret the meaning of stress in our lives. According to this theory, people experience lower levels of stress if they feel they are in control of a situation. The amount of control felt contributes to the degree of stress experienced. As we learned in Chapter 6, people with an internal locus of control hold the belief that control comes from one's own efforts; they see themselves as 'agents'. However, those with an external locus of control see themselves as 'victims'; they hold the belief that they are victims of circumstance.

Heider's (1958) *Attribution Theory*: According to this theory, humans are always trying to understand what is going on in the world around them, and to make sense of their own and others' behaviour. We have a tendency to look for causal explanations: we seek to understand why things happen and who is responsible for things happening. Typically, we will attribute the causes of events either to personality factors (dispositional attributions) or to external events (situational attributions). We are very prone to making a *Fundamental Attribution Error* (Ross 1977): we are more likely to perceive our own actions as arising from the situation, but others' actions as arising from their personality or disposition. So, for example, we might think 'Jenny failed that exam because she is lazy and doesn't study hard enough' (a dispositional attribution), but conversely, think 'I failed that exam because the teacher did not given me the correct textbook to revise from' (a situational attribution).

These theories (self efficacy, learned helplessness, locus of control, and attribution theory) can help us to understand our patients' responses when they find themselves in a stress inducing situation, such as being ill or being in hospital.

Coping with stress

Action point

When you feel under stress, what are you most likely to do to try to feel better?

You may have identified a number of behaviours which are likely to be helpful, such as going for a walk, and some which are unlikely to help in the long term, such as increasing alcohol use or driving aggressively. How do your patients cope with stress? If they are in hospital there may be a limited number of avenues for the release of their emotions. Essentially, however, the ways in which we deal with (i.e. try to reduce) stress will depend, in part, upon our belief systems and the success of previous coping strategies, and can be considered under three broad headings: Problem or task focused strategies, emotion focused strategies, and avoidant strategies.

Problem focused strategies: dealing with the stimulus

These strategies rely on taking direct action to remove the source of stress. This will involve:

- defining the problem;
- working out alternative solutions;
- weighing up the costs and benefits of these;
- implementing the chosen solution.

Because these strategies involve taking control of the situation, they may have the most positive outcome. However, there are some stressors that we simply cannot remove, and illness is often one such stressor. It may be that we have to help our patients to develop their emotion focused strategies to help them deal with the effects of their stressful situation.

Emotion focused strategies: dealing with the response

These strategies aim to address and reduce the negative effects of stress on our physiological functioning, behaviour, thoughts and emotions. They might include relaxation techniques, use of complementary therapies, or engaging in exercise. Often the most effective strategy is to enlist social support and to talk over the situation that is causing us stress. This can have the effect of seeing the problem in a new light (cognitive re-appraisal) as well as experiencing emotional unburdening or catharsis. As carers, we can contribute to the social support function by making time to listen to our patients' concerns, and in facilitating emotional expression, as we have noted in Chapters 5 and 6.

It should be noted that problem focused and emotion focused strategies are not mutually exclusive; for example, we might seek to improve our coping skills by training in assertiveness so that we are able to communicate our needs to others in a calm and consistent way. This is an emotion focused strategy, but it might also have the effect of removing a stressor from our lives. For example, if we learn to be able to say 'no' when our boss makes yet another unreasonable demand, this might in turn stop the boss from making unreasonable demands in the future (and thus remove the problem).

A third way of responding to stress is to try to avoid it. This involves minimising it or pretending it does not exist, and trying not to think about it. This strategy is generally thought to be the least effective of the three, although denial does have a role to play in certain phases of an illness experience (Eysenck 2009).

In this section, we have explored some theories underpinning human emotion, with particular reference to stress and anxiety, as such experiences are likely to be common during ill health and hospitalisation. Such knowledge should help us to recognise when someone is under stress and to respond from an informed perspective. We now consider some aspects of psychological knowledge that can help us in our information sharing role. We consider specifically memory and learning.

Knowledge for informational care

Memory

To be effective in informational care, a rudimentary knowledge of memory processes is important. Human memory involves three basic processes: *encoding*, whereby new material is presented to the senses; *storage*, whereby some or all of this new material is stored in the memory and is thus available to be accessed at a later times; and *retrieval*, which is the process of accessing and recovering stored material from memory.

It is thought that encoded material can be stored in a number of ways. First, a sensory store can hold information presented to the senses for a very short time only (up to a few seconds), and in the same medium as that in which it was presented (thus auditory material will be held in an echoic store; visual material in an iconic store). Short-term storage can hold a limited amount of material (7 +/–5 items such as words or numbers) for a short-time duration (around 2 minutes, unless it is actively rehearsed, such as by repeating a telephone number over and over to oneself); however this storage is very susceptible to disruption or interruption. More recently, the notion of short-term memory has been replaced with the idea of a 'working memory' that comprises several processing mechanisms and holds the information that an individual is consciously dealing with at any one time.

Long-term storage relies on many factors including efficient *mnemonics* (methods of organising information in meaningful ways) and imagery. Theoretically it has infinite capacity and can hold material indefinitely, and material from short-term memory may pass into long-term storage through rehearsal. However, just because material has been stored does not mean that we can retrieve it; what we may think of as 'forgetting' may actually be a failure to access and retrieve it from storage. Other theories of forgetting include:

- *Trace decay* (the idea that learning leaves a trace in the brain that gradually weakens or fades over time, especially if it is not used).
- *Displacement* (the idea that new learning will displace what is already stored).
- *Interference* (the idea that forgetting increases over time because there is increasing competition and interference from other information). Interference can be proactive – where information already stored interferes with the storage of new information – and retroactive – where information learned later interferes with the recall of previously stored information.
- *Repression*. This is based on Freud's idea that we are motivated to remove difficult or painful thoughts from our conscious mind (and push them into the unconscious), as a way of coping. This mechanism may have a part to play in explaining post-traumatic stress disorder, where people who have experienced a traumatic event display avoidance and numbing so as to minimise distressing thoughts about the event.

We also have a tendency to process and reconstruct events in an attempt to make sense of them, and this can lead to mis-remembering. An example of this is when we are asked leading or misleading questions, as demonstrated by Loftus and Palmer (1974) in their studies of eyewitness testimony. If, for example, when reporting a car accident to the police we are asked 'how fast was the car travelling' rather than 'at what speed was the car travelling' we may be inclined to give an over-estimate of speed, because of the inclusion of the word 'fast'. Hence we need to be careful in how we word our questions to patients; if we ask someone how 'severe' their pain is, for example, we may be prompting them to experience it as more severe than it actually is.

Primacy and recency effects

There is a tendency for people to remember best the information that is presented either early on (primacy effect) or at the end (recency effect) of a piece of communication, at which times it has the greatest impact. They therefore fail to recall much of the material presented in the middle of a piece of communication. This tendency is relevant also to impression formation, when our first impressions of people often make the greatest impact.

Action point

What does this all have to do with informational care? What principles of memory should we hold in mind when imparting information to our patients?

While there is no definitive understanding of all the processes involved in memory and forgetting (or failing to retrieve information from memory), awareness of these theories and principles will be important when we are providing information and also when we are asking people for information. It will perhaps help us to remember the principles of information giving that we outlined in Chapter 6: finding out the patient's experience, expectations, beliefs and understandings; giving specific rather than general information; stressing important content and repeating it as required; giving important information first and repeating it last; providing back up material for later reference, and providing the opportunity for the patient to ask us questions. It will perhaps also help to reduce our annoyance when information we know we have given appears not to have been remembered.

Learning

As we discovered in Chapter 2, theories of human learning largely arose from the work of the Behaviourist Psychologists Pavlov (1849–1936) and Skinner (1904–1990) and of the Social Learning theorist Bandura (1925 –). Behaviourists were seeking scientific principles to explain connections between actions and events and individuals' response to these events. They concluded that all behaviour occurs as a result of learning.

Action point

Either from your previous knowledge, or memory, or by revisiting Chapter 2, list three major theories of learning, and their key principles.

Pavlov's work gave rise to *classical conditioning*, and can be explained as 'learning by association'. Hence we form new associations (and thus learn new things) by connecting new environmental stimuli and our responses to those stimuli.

Skinner's theory of *operant conditioning* studied how such associations between stimuli and responses were made, and the theory could be described as 'learning by consequences', such that when behaviour receives positive reinforcement it is likely to be repeated. Hence, we learn to behave in a way that is likely to have positive consequences.

Bandura's *social learning theory* is an extension of these early theories of learning, and can be described as 'learning by observation'; especially from people we consider to be role models (we outlined the importance of role models in encouraging psychological care in Chapter 6).

Understanding the ways in which people learn (both patients and ourselves as carers) can be helpful in psychological care delivery. Understanding that a patient has had a bad experience of health care in the past (and perhaps might associate this with their current health care experience) might help to explain behaviour that could otherwise be perceived as 'difficult'. Reinforcement, by, for example, using minimal prompts (nods, smiles) and making time and space to listen to patients can be critical in encouraging patients to continue to talk to us and share their concerns. Finally, if we are seeking to encourage specific behaviours, we should be mindful of our influence as role models of the desired behaviour.

Knowledge for relationship based care

Finally, in exploring psychological knowledge that underpins effective psychological caregiving, we turn our attention to relationship based care. According to Nolan *et al.* (2001), the elements of a satisfactory health care relationship need to be studied and defined, because 'caregiving can only be understood in the concept of a relationship' and 'even transient relationships [in health care] can give rise to an emotional connection' (Paget 2010: 25). However, according to Nolan *et al.* (2001), the 'relationships that practitioners form with patients . . . have not generally been explored and taught explicitly'. So, what might we need to know, in order to understand the relationships our patients are forming with us and us with them? In this section we outline attachment theory and the concepts of transference and counter-transference and consider their relevance to relationship formation and maintenance and to psychological care.

Attachment theory

Attachment is essential to survival; as newborn babies we are driven to attach ourselves to other humans in order to satisfy our physiological needs. But attachment is about much more than just satisfying dietary needs and ensuring physical safety. In a series of now classic psychological experiments, Harlow (1958) noticed that a baby monkey raised on a bare wire-mesh cage floor 'survives with difficulty, if at all, during the first five days of life. If a wire-mesh cone is introduced, the baby does better; and, if the cone is covered with terry cloth, husky, healthy, happy babies evolve'. Hypothesising that something other than simply the provision of food was required for the monkey babies to survive, Harlow and colleagues built a surrogate 'mother' from a block of wood covered with sponge and soft cotton cloth, which was able to provide warmth from a light bulb. A second surrogate mother made of wire was able to dispense milk from an artificial teat. Harlow recorded the length of time baby monkeys spent with each of these surrogates and showed that much more time was spent clinging to the soft, warm 'mother' than to the wire lactating 'mother'. He concluded that 'contact comfort is a variable of overwhelming importance in the development of affectional response, whereas lactation is a variable of 'negligible importance' and that 'Certainly, man cannot live by milk alone'. Relationships are clearly important to survival, at least in monkeys. But what of humans?

Observational studies conducted by James and Joyce Robertson in the 1950s and 1960s of young children separated from their parents (such as was commonplace at the time when children or their parents were admitted to hospital) showed that such children would go through a series of stages in their behaviour. Initially, they would *protest* at the separation by crying, clinging, and frantically searching for the attachment figure. Subsequently, a *despair* stage developed, where the child seemed to have given up hope of the attachment figure ever returning, and became withdrawn and quiet. This was often interpreted by carers as evidence that the child was 'settling down'. In fact this was a precursor to the *detachment* phase in which the child transferred his or her interest to other people and the environment. However, when the attachment figure returned, the child showed little interest, almost as though punishing them for leaving. These landmark studies (see http://www.robertsonfilms.info/useful_links.htm) paved the way for John Bowlby (1907–1990), a British psychologist and psychiatrist, to explore the ways in which humans make emotional attachments with one another. Bowlby (1969) was able to show that when children experience security and comfort from a caregiver, they form an attachment bond to that person (attachment figure). He also demonstrated that children normally have a hierarchy of preferred attachment figures, and will seek out the primary attachment figure (usually but not always a parent, especially the mother) when they are distressed, seeking proximity and protesting if this person is unavailable. The primary attachment figure serves as a secure base from which to explore the world. Bowlby also showed that the nature of the attachments we make as babies and infants can have a profound effect on our subsequent development and capacity to form relationships, both as children and in adult life. Furthermore, our attachment experiences will impact on our mental health in adulthood.

Developing this work, Ainsworth and Bell (1970) showed that the nature of the attachments formed in infancy would have implications for later development (and, we can hypothesise, into adult life). In their classic 'strange situation' experiment, infants aged between 12 and 18 months were observed though a one-way mirror playing happily with a parent. After a short time, a stranger entered the room, and after another short period of time, the parent left the room, leaving the child and stranger alone. Subsequent steps in the experiment involved leaving the child alone; the stranger returning, the parent returning, and finally the stranger leaving. Observing for separation anxiety, stranger anxiety, and the reaction of the child when reunited with its parent, Ainsworth and Bell concluded that children had by this age formed either secure or insecure attachments with their parent, which determined how they reacted when left with a stranger or alone, and how they reacted when reunited with the parent. Most children behaved in the way predicted by Bowlby: they become upset when the parent left the room, but actively sought out the parent on their return, and appeared comforted by their return. However, others did not behave in this way, and it was hypothesised that the children who appeared insecure in the strange situation experiment had parents who were insensitive to their needs, or who were inconsistent or rejecting in the care they provided (Fraley 2010). Insecure attachment was assumed from any of three observed patterns of behaviour – ambivalent, avoidant or disorganised. Those with an ambivalent attachment style (possibly learned through having a parent who responds inconsistently and insensitively) would intensify their attachment behaviours in order to get a response, by, for example, clinging, crying or attention seeking. Those with an avoidant attachment style, perhaps learned through having a rejecting or controlling attachment figure, would eventually cease attachment behaviours and become undemanding, compliant and self-sufficient. Finally, those with a disorganised attachment style (perhaps as a result of having had an abusive or unresponsive caregiver) would learn that no attachment behaviour would bring care and comfort, and so would attempt to control a frightening world by avoiding attachment seeking.

According to Golding (2007) there can be serious consequences of insecure attachment upon the cognitive, behavioural, social and emotional development of children. These consequences can include behaviour such as anger, violence, blaming others, lying, stealing and cruelty. Social effects can include poor relationships with peers; being demanding and clingy; lacking affection with carers; and indiscriminate affection with strangers. Emotionally, there may be resentment; fear and shame. But do these effects last into adulthood, and if so, how can knowing about attachment styles help us in delivering good psychological care to our patients?

Attachment and adults

According to Fraley (2010), it is likely that similar processes are in operation between adults in personal relationships as with parent–child attachments. Indeed, Bowlby showed that the effects of early bonding and attachment experiences lasted into adult life and could determine the nature and security of adult interpersonal relationships and even predict adult mental health problems. Bowlby believed that it was during attachment formation in infancy that a child develops expectations and beliefs about relationships generally. Thus, a securely attached child (and later, adult) will have a belief that others are dependable and trustworthy, and will thus expect this in adult relationships. In studies, adults who had secure romantic relationships tended to remember their childhood relationships with parents as affectionate and caring (Fraley 2010). Of course, adverse experiences in later relationships can challenge this belief system, but the foundations are likely to be set.

Adult attachment has begun to receive serious attention during the past thirty years, with some researchers hypothesising that if attachment to others in adulthood has the same functions as in infancy (such as providing a secure base and meeting emotional and comfort needs), then it is likely that the same patterns of secure and insecure attachments are probably in operation too, and this has been verified by researchers such as Brennan, Clark and Shaver (1998). In terms of romantic relationships, Brennan *et al.* found that insecurely attached adults worried that their partners may not be available or responsive to them, yet at the same time felt unable to rely on or open up to others. Furthermore, securely attached adults are more likely than insecure adults to seek support when distressed (Fraley 2010). These features may be replicated in any adult relationships. In conclusion, it seems that the attachment system of infancy continues to influence behaviour, thought, and feeling in adulthood (Fraley 2010). So as carers, we may witness patterns of behaviour in our patients indicating secure or insecure attachment styles that might have an impact on the kinds of relationships they form with us and us with them.

Transference and counter-transference

A related and important factor in understanding therapeutic relationships is the concept of transference and its opposite concept counter-transference. Originating with Freud, transference means 'a bridge', and it is thought to be closely linked to early attachments. It can be described as the unconscious process of bringing and transferring feelings that originated in other relationships into current relationships. A key feature is that feelings and behaviours linked to more than one person can transfer from one relationship to another regardless of gender or context (Jones 2005). Hence, patterns of relationships formed during early development are repeated in the present. Transference can be positive or negative or a mixture; positive transference might manifest itself in expressions of love or admiration, while negative transference can result in hostility or even hatred. *Counter-transference* is a response to transference, influenced by the features of that particular transference.

An understanding of both concepts is critical in understanding relationships in health care, in part because these relationships are rarely emotionally neutral and are thus likely to evoke strong transferences and counter-transferences (Jones 2005). For example, patients are often dependent on nurses and other health professionals to take care of them when they are ill, and they may transfer feelings of being dependent on a parent when they were a child. As pointed out by de Raeve (2010: 59), 'nurses . . . are common recipients of maternal transference from patients'. This may, for example, manifest itself in the patient being excessively clingy or demanding. Health care providers, in response, might, for example, respond to such dependency behaviours in ways that evoke their own experiences of caring for their own children or other dependents. Jones (2005) suggests a number of examples of how transference (both positive and negative) and counter-transference may operate in the nurse–patient relationship. These include strong feelings of affection or dislike; desires to please or avoid, over- or under-involvement, feelings of comfort or discomfort with the other person. A basic understanding of how these feelings might have arisen can help us as health carers to identify difficulties and manage relationships more effectively.

Summary

One overriding difficulty in identifying an appropriate body of knowledge that will facilitate the delivery of psychological care is concerned with the nature of psychological knowledge itself. It is clear that many psychological concepts have become absorbed into everyday life and language. Danziger (1990, 1997), in his studies of the history of psychology and its impact in everyday life, has described the process through which psychology established itself as an applied science, and through which psychologists were able to claim special expertise. Eventually, psychological knowledge became re-incorporated into the everyday world. It is often difficult, then, to recognise psychological concepts as discrete topics worthy of academic study. Carers may well discuss phenomena such as attachment, thinking, learning or emotions in relation to patient care, with little awareness of the complexities of these phenomena and the knowledge base that underpins them. It is perhaps not surprising, then, that decisions about what psychological knowledge is relevant to caring, about how it should be taught, and about how it should be made relevant to practice, and in particular to the delivery of psychological care, have been so apparently diverse and arbitrary.

Despite these challenges, in this chapter, we have interrogated the knowledge base of psychology for information that might support our personal qualities and skills and help us in our endeavours as psychological caregivers. We have identified social psychological knowledge such as social perception, impression formation, stereotypes, attitudes and prejudice that can support our psychological assessment and monitoring skills; we have explored knowledge around emotion and stress that might help us to deliver more effective emotional care; we have sought out knowledge around memory and learning that could support informational care; and finally we have considered the concepts of attachment, transference and counter-transference in helping us develop effective interpersonal relationships within our practice. Perhaps we can now challenge Biley's statement that opened this chapter, and conclude that although it is not *just* knowledge that makes a difference in health care practice, relevant scientific and specifically psychological knowledge can enhance and support the qualities and skills needed to deliver effective psychological care.

8   Psychological care in context

> People are confident that the care environment meets their needs and preferences.
>
> (Department of Health 2010: 7)

Introduction

Thus far, we have discussed psychological needs and care in very general terms, as they might apply to any person with ill health in almost any context. In this chapter, we present and discuss psychological care delivery in a range of health care contexts, including medical and surgical wards, general practice, care of older people, learning disability settings, and in loss and bereavement. Two further case studies describe the process of referral to specialist psychological services, to illustrate the judgements that carers have to make about when and to whom such referrals might be made, and the communication processes needed to facilitate smooth referral experiences.

The chapter draws on case studies of psychological needs and care in these contexts, and in this way allows consideration of the role of context, culture and environment in identifying and responding to psychological needs. While these case studies are based on real people and situations, they have been anonymised, with all identifying details removed or altered. Following each case study, we will consider the patient's psychological needs and the psychological care they might require. It is acknowledged that these case studies do not represent the entire range of care experiences that the reader of this book might encounter, but it is hoped that the common strategies can be applied to a wide range of care settings and clinical situations, encouraging the carer to focus explicitly on the psychological needs of patients alongside their physical and other care needs. Furthermore, there is no attempt to consider every possible aspect of psychological care that might be relevant in each case; rather an example or two have been selected as the focus for each case study.

In reading the case studies and thinking about which aspects of psychological care might be relevant, you might like to refer back to Chapter 4 of this book, in which we identified the core elements of psychological care and the prerequisites for effective psychological care delivery.

Action point

After you have read each case study, jot down your immediate responses to the following questions:

- How might this particular care environment have impacted on the patient's psychological needs?
- What psychological care skills were used or could have been used?
- What psychological knowledge was helpful or might have been helpful in this particular case?
- Were there any barriers to providing psychological care, and if so, how might they have been overcome?

Case study 1: Psychological care in a medical assessment unit

Mrs Mary Riley, aged 70, was admitted to the Medical Assessment Unit following a fall and a period of confusion, as reported by her daughter; this confusion was found to be due to a urinary tract infection. Basic nursing observations of vital signs were recorded on admission, and medical and social histories were taken. Subsequently, care plans were drawn up for falls and dietary intake (as her daughter was concerned she was not eating enough). Physiotherapists helped Mrs Riley with mobility by providing her with a new walking frame which was better suited to her height and posture than her old one. Occupational therapists assessed her fine motor skills to see how well she managed independently with the activities of daily living.

A registered mental health nurse then assessed her cognitive ability and mental capacity by carrying out a 'Mini Mental State Examination' (MMSE), and she scored 24, indicating a very mild degree of cognitive impairment.

Mrs Riley relied heavily on her daughter's visits and became anxious when she didn't know where her daughter was, so the staff assured her frequently that her daughter would be there at visiting times. If she wanted to speak to her daughter at other times, staff generally let Mrs Riley use the ward phone.

After a week's course of antibiotics the doctors deemed Mrs Riley medically fit for discharge. However, her social assessment suggested that she would not be safe to return home with her existing care package, as she was finding it difficult to cope with carers calling to assist only twice a day. It was decided that her care package should be increased with the aim of helping to meet her hygiene and mobility needs and general ability to cope at home. As it took time to set up this new care package, Mrs Riley's discharge was delayed by 4 weeks.

Mrs Riley was keen to go home and live independently, but her confusion and memory problems meant that she could not remember how long she had been in hospital and she seemed content to remain there. However, when she was told the delay was to arrange extra help for her at home, she became angry and refused to believe that she needed help and was coping fine on her own. Even with her daughter trying to persuade her it was for the best she told her she was being ridiculous. Otherwise Mrs Riley was quite content, loved to talk, and let the nurses know if another patient needed help if they could not get to the call buzzer.

Key areas of psychological care for Mrs Riley

Mrs Riley is in an unfamiliar environment and is likely to be anxious about where she is and what is happening to her. She seems to be missing her daughter to whom she is clearly close and on whom she perhaps relies for support and information. Her level of confusion may mean that her information needs are not always being met, and she may need regular and frequent reminders about what is happening and why. However, her MMSE score (Folstein and Folstein 1975) showed only a mild level of impairment, which could perhaps be attributed to confusion arising from her urinary tract infection. Once this is treated, her confusion may lessen. She is likely to need time to express her emotions of anxiety and anger and this can to some extent be provided during physical care activities, but extra time may be needed as she loves to talk and this need should be met if possible. The small act of allowing her access to the ward phone has been effective in allaying some of her anxieties about where her daughter is, but Mrs Riley will benefit from developing a meaningful and trusting relationship with (ideally) one or a small number of carers while she is waiting to be discharged. Mrs Riley clearly enjoys being helpful to others and could perhaps be given other simple ward tasks to undertake, to boost her self esteem and sense of value.

It will be helpful if Mrs Riley's carers understand something of the ageing process and the psychological needs of the older person. Losses and changes in older age, such as retirement, bereavement and the loss of a significant role in society, can all challenge psychological well-being, particularly as they are often seen in a negative light by the older person and those around them (Victor 2010). In addition to these general experiences, Mrs Riley has recently experienced a number of other losses such as regular contact with her daughter, her familiar home environment, deteriorating memory, and reduced mobility following her fall. Older people are thought to be particularly vulnerable to experiencing multiple negative events and they may have fewer resources to cope (Victor 2010). Resilience, or 'responding positively to adversity' (Hildon cited in Victor: 95) is seen as an attribute of successful ageing, and is a protective factor in older age. However, resilience may involve developing new coping strategies to compensate for failings, such as effective memory aids, so Mrs Riley may find it helpful to develop a notebook or calendar reminder system while she is in hospital that she can continue once she is home. It is important also to note that neither cognitive decline nor deterioration in well being are inevitable in older age; in fact, some studies have shown that the presumption of irreversible cognitive decline is a stereotype and oversimplification, and in fact the majority of older people are in good psychological health (Victor 2010). However, it should be noted that depression is very common in older age, and that it often goes undiagnosed or misdiagnosed as the early stages of dementia, so it will be important to assess and monitor Mrs Riley's mood and to report any changes in case a referral to mental health specialists is required.

In Mrs Riley's case, we have attempted to illustrate how the key psychological principles of informational care, emotional care, using small acts, observation skills, and relationship building might be used in enhancing her psychological well being.

Case study 2: Psychological care in the surgical ward

Miss Claire Miller, aged 27, was admitted to the surgical ward with generalised abdominal pain. She had given birth to a healthy baby nine months previously, following a difficult pregnancy, during which she had needed a surgical procedure to treat a serious medical problem. The surgery was successful, although Claire needed to stay in the intensive therapy unit (ITU) for a few days and required regular analgesia for severe pain. Despite being so unwell, Claire subsequently had a normal birth and returned home. Claire lived alone with her baby, as the baby's father had not felt ready to be tied down. Her parents lived abroad and were unable to visit often, although she had a supportive network of friends.

Claire had had several admissions to hospital since surgery complaining of abdominal pain, but no physical abnormalities had been found that could account for her pain. On her latest admission, she had made repeated requests to the staff for more complex investigations such as scans and a laparoscopy (whereby an incision is made in the abdomen to permit abdominal structures to be seen via a small camera and sometimes, to carry out minor surgical procedures), as she was sure there was something physically wrong, and she continued to be distressed and complaining of pain. Her doctors felt that if they carried out these tests to rule out any abnormalities, she would then be reassured that nothing was wrong. If she continued to experience pain, then this could be explained as psychological in nature, perhaps as a result of her bad experiences during pregnancy and in ITU, and thus a referral could be made to appropriate services such as counselling. In fact, Claire's test results showed no abnormalities, and when the possibility of a psychological explanation was broached with her she agreed that she had felt anxious since her traumatic pregnancy, and was finding it difficult to cope alone with her young baby.

Key areas of psychological care for Claire

Claire seems to be experiencing some strong emotions associated with her pain experience and apparent absence of a clear physical explanation. It is believed that there is always a psychological aspect of pain, and in particular the emotions of anxiety, anger, helplessness, and depression are common, with anxiety most often associated with acute pain and depression with chronic pain (Davies 2000). Anxiety in response to pain is often associated with uncertainty about what the pain means and whether it will ever go away, and can lead to catastrophic thinking: fearing the worst will happen or has already happened. The unpleasant symptoms of anxiety can exacerbate pain symptoms, and catastrophising can lead to higher levels of pain and resulting disability (Davis 2000).

Exploring a patient's responses using emotional care skills is often the best way to determine the kind of interventions that will be most helpful. When given the opportunity to talk about how she felt, Claire understood that the problem she had experienced during pregnancy was rare and could not help feeling 'why me?' She felt sure that her pain meant she had sustained some permanent damage and that she would never be well again. She worried that she would be unable to continue to care for her baby and felt angry that staff did not believe she was in pain. Over the days that Claire was undergoing tests and waiting for the results, her carers were able to express unconditional positive regard, and using counselling skills, were able to show Claire that she was a valued human being who was deserving of their time and attention. They also showed that they understood the pain experience was real for her.

Over time, Claire was able to express her sadness that the baby's father had rejected her, also her anger that she was left to cope with a young baby on her own. While her pain was real, she was able to acknowledge that perhaps coming into hospital for investigations met some of her needs for care and attention that were not being met elsewhere. Staff helped Claire to monitor her pain by using a visual analogue scale and Claire was pleased to note that her rating of pain severity reduced over the few days she was in hospital. Simply being given the information that there was no medical reason why she should continue to be in pain helped Claire to reappraise and reframe her experience and this contributed to a reduction in both pain and anxiety. The staff also knew that distraction could often help in reducing pain and anxiety, and encouraged Claire to listen to her favourite music on her headphones whenever she felt particularly worried. They also gave her a website address where she could download some relaxation exercises to listen to when she felt particularly worried. Claire left hospital after a few days, not completely pain free but feeling more positive about her health and ability to cope in the future.

In Claire's case, we have illustrated how the key psychological principles of observation, empathy, unconditional positive regard, emotional care, informational care, and counselling skills might be used in enhancing her psychological well being.

Case study 3: Psychological care in General Practice

Mr Joseph Magwenzi, aged 52, was born in Zimbabwe but had lived in Birmingham for 11 years since moving to England to look for work. He lived in a rented flat with his female partner, and had lost touch with his three grown-up children; he was unsure of their whereabouts. He no longer had contact with his family in Zimbabwe.

Three years ago Joseph was taken by his partner to the local hospital's accident and emergency department complaining of a severe cough and feeling generally unwell. He was admitted to hospital where tests revealed that his cough was caused by tuberculosis (TB). Further investigations showed that he was HIV positive (that is, he was infected with the human immunodeficiency virus which causes AIDS [acquired immune-deficiency syndrome] and is transmitted via blood to blood or sexual contact. Joseph was initially shocked at both these diagnoses, although he was relieved to have an explanation for his symptoms. Joseph was a very co-operative patient, taking all prescribed medication and attending all routine GP and outpatient clinic appointments.

During one such routine appointment at the GP surgery, he was seen by a medical student who talked to him about living with a chronic illness. Joseph said that he was shocked to have received the HIV diagnosis, but believed he had contracted it when he was working for the council, cleaning public toilets, and that it was God's will. The medical student was unsure if he really understood the nature of his illness, nor how it was contracted and transmitted, and was concerned for the sexual health of his female partner. The student passed her concerns on to the GP who was surprised, having assumed that Joseph would have had everything explained to him very thoroughly at the hospital HIV clinic. The GP said he would check out Joseph's knowledge next time he saw him.

Key areas of psychological care for Joseph

Joseph clearly has unmet information needs as his misunderstanding of the nature and cause of HIV was potentially placing not only himself but also his partner at risk. Because he was attending scheduled appointments it is perhaps unsurprising that this crucial fact had been missed in the busy GP practice. The fact that he was considered to be a 'compliant' patient, apparently doing everything he had been advised to do by his health care team, might have meant that assumptions were made about his level of understanding without checking these out in reality.

It is likely, given his extreme misunderstanding of how HIV is acquired, that Joseph is also unaware that a HIV infection will eventually become full blown AIDS, which places the individual at increased risk of other infections and cancers, and ultimately leads to death. He therefore may not have had the opportunity to discuss with anyone the implications of a terminal diagnosis. It is possible also that he may have confused symptoms of HIV with symptoms of TB, such as tiredness or weight loss.

Careful inter-professional communication between the GP practice and the specialist out-patient clinic team should ensure that this information lapse is rectified and that Joseph and his partner are fully informed about the risks to their individual physical and sexual health. Sensitivity will be required in addressing sexual matters with the couple, particularly in relation to their cultural and religious values and beliefs. We do not know whether Joseph or his partner is responsible for transmitting this infection to the other, or if one of them has possibly acquired it via sexual contact with a third party, or if it has been acquired, for example, via injecting drugs. It is likely that Joseph and his partner would benefit from referral to a specialist service in this respect, especially one that has a focus on cross-cultural issues.

In Joseph's case, we have aimed to illustrate how the key psychological principles of social perception, informational care, communication skills, and referral skills might be used in enhancing his psychological (and indeed physical) wellbeing.

Case study 4: Psychological care in the nursing home

Mrs Gladys Evans is an 89-year-old widow who is currently living in a specialist nursing home for people suffering from dementia. She was diagnosed over 10 years ago with Alzheimer's disease. Mrs Evans has two married sons who are themselves in their 60s, and unable to visit often. Her grandchildren and great grandchildren visit only rarely and Mrs Evans does not appear to know who they are when they visit.

Over the past year she has lost much of her ability to communicate through spoken language. She is, however, able to express some of her needs, likes, and dislikes through repeating single words and through her facial expressions, gestures, and non-verbal expressions (such as shouting and crying). Some of these expressions of distress are challenging to her carers, who sometimes struggle to understand what she needs. Mrs Evans also spends considerable time wandering around the home, sometimes getting lost and disturbing other residents' belongings. She is disoriented as to time and therefore wanders at any time of the day or night. Staff are concerned that Mrs Evans will become exhausted by her excessive wanderings and apparent distress and have asked that she be prescribed medication to help her to settle and achieve a more regular sleep–wake pattern.

Key areas of psychological care for Mrs Evans

The term 'dementia' describes a syndrome which can be caused by a number of illnesses (including Alzheimer's disease) in which there is progressive decline in multiple areas of function including memory, motor function, recognition, language, executive function, planning, and sequencing (Department of Health 2009, 2010b). As we have previously noted, cognitive decline is not inevitable in older age, but the prevalence of dementia does increase as age rises, affecting around 30 per cent of the population who are aged over 95. In addition to general knowledge about ageing, it is crucial that carers in this setting have a clear understanding of the diagnosis and types of dementia, its manifestations, and effective interventions.

One issue identified within the Department of Health's (2009, 2010b) National Strategy for Dementia was the over-prescription of antipsychotic medication for people with dementia. It estimated that there are around 180,000 people with dementia on antipsychotic (major tranquillising) drugs, but that this is only beneficial for around a third of these people, and that there are 1800 excess deaths per year as a result of their prescription. While the carers' requests for such medication were clearly made in Mrs Evans' best interests, it would be important for them to have an understanding of psychologically driven alternatives to medication.

One such alternative could be the use of elements of dementia care mapping, which will help with the assessment and monitoring of Mrs Evans' psychological needs and support emotional care delivery. Dementia care mapping is an observation tool designed at Bradford University, based on Kitwood's (1997) work on person-centered care (http://www.brad.ac.uk/health/dementia/DementiaCareMapping). Person-centred care in dementia can be defined as care that 'values all people regardless of age and health status, is individualized, emphasizes the perspective of the person with dementia, and stresses the importance of relationships' (Brooker 2004: 11). Dementia care mapping uses these values to examine behaviour, communication and care needs from the perspective of the person with dementia (Brooker 2005). When undertaken formally, trained 'mappers' work in pairs, spending a set time period such as six hours observing up to five people and events around them in a given communal care area. Every five minutes, mappers code the behaviour of the people they are observing according to a checklist, and score whether it is indicative of well-being or ill-being. Well-being, according to Kitwood, is directly related to the quality of care delivered. Mappers also record personal detractions (staff behaviours that could undermine personhood) and positive events (that enhance personhood). Afterwards, the mappers analyse the data and provide feedback to staff as a means of improving care wherever possible.

While it is unlikely that care settings for people with dementia will employ many if any trained care mappers, the fact that the process uses a combination of empathy and observational skills (Kitwood 1997) means that the basic skills and strategies could be developed by carers to enhance their psychological care delivery in this context. In Mrs Evans's case, her wandering behaviour and expressions of distress could perhaps be observed and understood as feeling lost and frightened in a strange environment, particularly as her short-term memory is likely to be poor (see Chapter 7). She may be unable to retain information and thus need constant reminders of where she is and what is happening around her.

Related to these strategies, carers may find that using elements of validation therapy could enhance Mrs Evans's psychological well being. Validation therapy was developed as a way of communicating effectively with older adults with dementia, based on non-judgemental respect and empathy and a belief that people are unique and valuable (Feil 1991). It is aimed at building trusting relationships with carers, reducing anxiety and promoting dignity.

The validation approach assumes that there is a reason for the behaviour of older people and while the reason may not be immediately obvious, careful observation may reveal triggers and patterns that can help to explain it. A further principle is that emotions are real, even if the patient's understanding of the situation is flawed due to cognitive decline. For example, Mrs Evans was often observed to be calling out 'Mama' in the course of her wanderings around the nursing home, with facial expressions indicative of fear. Clearly in reality, Mrs Evans could not have a living mother, and it may be thought best to try to distract her from her disorientation and perhaps gently remind her that she is in the residential home, rather than at home with her mother. However, in validation therapy, rather than distract or dismiss behaviours in this way, carers aim to acknowledge that the patient's feelings are real (i.e. validate them) and accept that even though their expression might be out of keeping with the generally accepted reality, they should be identified and respected as a genuine expression of how that person feels at that time. In this case, the painful feelings of anxiety or fear expressed by Mrs Evans may be because she feels lost in her environment. Present emotions can trigger similar emotions experienced in the past, even in childhood, which may explain why she is anxiously seeking her mother for comfort and reassurance. Rather than focus on (or avoid) the search for 'Mama', the carer might instead focus on acknowledging the emotion and helping Mrs Evans to feel safe and secure in her current environment, perhaps modelling some elements of the 'mother' role that she appears to be missing.

In Mrs Evans's case, we have illustrated how the key psychological principles of observation, empathy, unconditional positive regard, informational care, emotional care, communication skills, relationship building and role modelling might be used to enhance her psychological well-being.

Case study 5: Psychological care in cancer

Mr Elliott Stevens, aged 28, is single and lives alone. His closest family members live several hours' drive away. After returning home from a bicycle ride, Elliott had noticed a small lump in his neck. He visited his GP who was unsure of the nature of the problem and referred him to a hospital specialist. The lump was thought to be a cyst, was drained, and Elliott was sent on his way with the full expectation that the problem would not recur. The lump reappeared three times, however, and on each occasion it was drained and Elliott was discharged with no follow-up. Losing faith in the medical profession, Elliot turned to Chinese acupuncture which offered some relief but did not prevent the lump from returning.

Eventually he was sent for surgery to remove the lump. When it was tested in the laboratory, it was found to be malignant and indicative of thyroid cancer, so Elliott was asked to return for surgery to remove the entire thyroid gland. The surgery to remove his thyroid gland had also caused damage to his parathyroid glands, a common consequence of this surgery. The parathyroid glands control the body's blood calcium levels. If they are not working properly, calcium levels can fall below normal, causing twitching and muscle spasms, so Elliott was prescribed calcium tablets in addition to the thyroxine that his body needed following removal of his thyroid gland. In hospital for 10 days, Elliott described this period as a 'rollercoaster nightmare' in which his calcium levels fluctuated widely and he experienced many unpleasant side effects.

This surgery was followed up with radioactive iodine treatment, which picks up and kills any remaining thyroid cancer cells wherever they are in the body, to prevent further spread. There is a small risk that radioactive iodine can cause other cancers in the future but it is believed that the benefits outweigh these risks.

Elliott was referred for support to the specialist endocrinology nurse who was able to act as an intermediary between him and the ward staff. After Elliott's treatment and discharge he experienced many complications including a bad response to the radio-active iodine and an apparently accidental overdose of calcium just after leaving hospital, which affected his balance and caused a sensation of pressure in his chest and blurred vision. He was readmitted to hospital as a medical emergency.

Key areas of psychological care for Elliott

Elliott needed considerable support during the post operative and subsequent period as changes were happening rapidly in his body as his calcium levels fluctuated. He has been told that if he remains well for five years his chances of a full recovery are very good; hence this five-year period is a time of great stress and uncertainty including worry about recurrence and other potential problems caused by the iodine treatment and calcium intake. Elliott also feels angry that several opportunities to identify the problem early on were missed and that he suffered unnecessarily. The opportunity to access counselling via the hospital's cancer centre remains open during this time as he experiences emotional as well as physical changes and concerns. In addition, the endocrine support nurse provides an invaluable source of information and support and is available at the end of the phone when Elliott needs to discuss and understand his regular blood test results. Elliott was also put in touch with a specialist UK-wide support group (the Butterfly Trust) which was started by someone who had experienced thyroid cancer and felt there was not enough support available. The Trust offers information, support and encouragement, and through this organisation, Elliott was able to talk to others with thyroid cancer by email and telephone contact; could seek advice via their helpline, and could request a 'buddy' to be on hand through the treatment process. This support has been invaluable as Elliot's family are unable to be with him during his recovery period. Two years post surgery, Elliott has recognised that he might benefit from being helped to express his anger and anxiety and feelings of being 'let down' by the medical and hospital system, and has engaged with a hospital-based counselling service.

While Elliott's information needs have generally been well met, his emotional care needs appear to have been less well catered for, and early opportunities to assess and monitor his psychological needs and facilitate emotional expression may have been missed. This case study illustrates how the key psychological care principles of assessment and monitoring, informational care, communication skills, self care, advocacy and referral might be used in conjunction with medical care to enhance his psychological wellbeing.

Psychological care in intellectual disabilities – loss and death

We present here two case studies that illustrate the psychological needs of two people whose physical health needs were compounded by their having intellectual disabilities and a number of needs in relation to loss, bereavement and death. Key principles for psychological care are discussed in relation to the continuum ranging from death and dying to responding to loss.

Case study 6: Laura Martin

Laura was 74, had an intellectual disability and poor communication skills, and had lived in care all her life, moving from large institutions to hostels and small homes, and eventually settling in a small bungalow with four other ladies. This bungalow was situated within a council estate in a small but busy town. From here the ladies enjoyed a full range of social activities and events within the local community.

Laura had suffered ill health for a short time and was eventually diagnosed with having advanced lung cancer, with a poor prognosis. Initially the bungalow care staff (all untrained young women with little or no experience of death or dying either personally or professionally) experienced a range of emotions: shock, confusion, sadness and uncertainty about what to expect and how to talk to Laura; self-doubt about how they would cope; and a profound sense of disbelief and denial as Laura did not look significantly unwell. Laura herself had an innate fear of hospitals and nurses and rarely complained of ill health.

Case study 7: John Brown

John is 50 years old and has diabetes, which is controlled by insulin. He lives with three other men who all have varying degrees of intellectual disabilities. Four months ago, one of the men died suddenly the week before Christmas. John did not go to the funeral because his father forbade it. John's mother had died some ten years previously and it transpired that John had never been told that she had died, but that she had simply been admitted to hospital. His father said this was because he wanted John to be pro-tected from the sadness of losing his mother. John had no photographs of his mother, and when he asked his father about her (which he frequently did) he was told that she was still in hospital having tests.

Since the death of his friend, John's behaviour had deteriorated. He sat for long periods of time crying in the deceased friend's bedroom, which was currently unoccupied but would shortly be allocated to someone else. Additionally, his diabetes was no longer under control and he needed frequent visits to the Out Patient clinic for his insulin levels to be monitored and for John and his carers to have continuing advice about the management of his diabetes. John became very agitated when faced with the prospect of these hospital visits, although he was always accompanied by a familiar carer from his home.

Services for people with intellectual disabilities are usually focused on helping people to live well with their disability rather than on dying well, so carers are often not familiar with the issues surrounding end of life care (Todd 2006). However, people with intellectual dis-abilities are living longer and well into older age, and will experience the range of health conditions often associated with increased longevity. Therefore it is important that carers develop a repertoire of skills alongside specialist services provided, for example, by pallia-tive care teams and hospice care services (Read and Morris 2009). Equally, they need an awareness of available services such as the 'hospice at home' schemes that are widely available based within local hospices, and local advocacy services to support the person in sensitive situations.

In Laura's case, local intellectual disabilities services, district nursing and palliative care services needed to become well integrated in order to provide holistic care and support to ensure that her individual needs were met; that she was at the centre of all decisions about her care; and that she maintained as much autonomy as possible throughout her palliative journey. Laura had communication difficulties, and it is often forgotten that people with cognitive and communication difficulties can and do experience strong and often painful emotions and indeed physical pain, but often lack the verbal repertoire to express this in comprehensible ways. Adequate assessments of pain, distress and symptom management and emotional care are crucial to effective care and support, and resources such as the DisDAT tool (Reynard *et al.* 2007) are welcomed. This is the only available comprehensive distress tool developed specifically for people with intellectual disabilities (www.mencap.org.uk/document.asp).

The emotional needs of people with an intellectual disability often remain neglected (Arthur 2003), for a variety of reasons, perhaps because of perceptions of their ability to express meaningful emotion; over-protectiveness by carers; or even carers' feelings of fear, inadequacy and uncertainty in how to deal with emotional distress (Read 2008). The psychological support needs inherent in dying and indeed the aftermath of death (bereavement) may often go unnoticed and subsequently unresolved for the person with an intellectual disability, even though they are seen as integral to holistic care and support. Often people with an intellectual disability experience disenfranchised grief (Doka 1989), as evidenced by John's experience. People with intellectual disabilities often live in the shadow of grief and are often deliberately excluded from the rituals around death because family and carers want to protect them from distress and the sad business of loss. Carers need to be mindful that death in the family affects all of the family; John's father had, though, been able to assert his need to grieve while John had been denied this right at the time. Consequently John missed his mother, felt this loss profoundly, but could not understand why she didn't visit him anymore. John was left trying to make sense of nonsense.

It is likely that his recent experience of a housemate dying had triggered John's unresolved grief, causing behaviour changes, and a likely response from his carers would be to make a referral to a behaviour therapist and to organise a medication review. In John's case, staff were unsure what to do because they wanted to help him, but were also sensitive to the family's (perhaps misguided) wish to protect John from further upset.

The key to unlocking these issues remained with helping his father to understand that John needed to be treated with openness and honesty, and supported to grieve for his mother and friend in socially acceptable ways. To resolve this dilemma staff met with John's father (with the support of a bereavement counsellor) and eventually his father gave permission for staff to explain to John what had happened to his mother (although he felt unable to talk with John about it himself). A process of grief work was then initiated, treating John as a competent adult at all times while exposing him gently to the reality of his mother's death. This included going to see the place where she was buried, choosing flowers, dressing for the occasion, taking flowers to the cemetery, and obtaining photos of his mother for John to display in his room. Such activities are all constructive and meaningful ways of commemorating the loss of a loved one. John's father was also invited to participate in these activities.

Death and dying are sensitive topics, and carers will also have support needs when a person they have cared for dies, as will the other people with intellectual disabilities who (in Laura's case) formed part of her 'family'. In these two case studies, we have shown how principles of informational care, observation, empathy, unconditional positive regard, emotional care, informational care, and small acts might be used in enhancing psychological well being. Additionally, clinical supervision, staff counselling services or generic counselling services may provide opportunities for the carers in these case scenarios to explore their feelings and seek the psychological support they require at this time.

Referring on: the role of other professionals in enhancing psychological care

Within several of the chapters of this book, we have noted that a key element of care delivery (and not just psychological care) is for carers to identify the limits of their knowledge and skill and to know when to seek further guidance or indeed to refer on for specialist psycho-logical support. The two remaining case studies in this chapter illustrate how a referral process might be instigated, and how specialist psychological interventions can be used to help.

Case study 8: Psychological care in obstetric services

Mrs Samantha Smith, aged 34 years, was referred to a clinical psychologist for psycho-logical therapy by her midwife, because she reported having experienced her last childbirth as traumatic and was struggling to manage antenatal contact with the maternity service now she was pregnant again. She was 16 weeks pregnant at the time of the referral, and her previous (first) child had been born 3 years earlier.

Her last experience of childbirth involved having a long attempt at a vaginal delivery, which then did not progress and an emergency caesarean section was performed. The baby was born healthy. During the labour, Samantha had become so exhausted, frightened and felt in so much pain that she felt unable to speak and so was unable to communicate her wishes. Normally someone who is assertive and quick to challenge authority, Samantha found she was unable to advocate for herself – as well as anger with maternity staff, she also felt resentment towards her mother and partner for not refusing some procedures on her behalf and for not questioning staff. She was angry that she had been inconsistently consulted about even quite invasive procedures e.g. a catheter was put in place without discussion with her, yet it was judged that she was able to think clearly enough to sign a consent form for a caesarean section. She also believed that a number of internal examinations (to check on progress and dilation) had been unnecessary (partly confirmed from discussion with midwives and an obstetrician later), and brusque as well as very painful. She described her overall experience in the hospital as being 'treated like a piece of meat'.

During one stage, Samantha believed that she would not survive (something she fully realised when she got home, as she found herself walking through each room of her house not having expected to ever see it again). This was more frightening for her a bit later rather than during labour, as she described feeling so overwhelmed at that stage that she welcomed death to escape everything. This was also a source of difficult feelings for her later, as she felt guilty about her lack of thought about the baby at that point. The emergency caesarean was experienced as an immediate 'relief' to Samantha (in contrast to many women for whom it is the traumatic element) compared to what had happened up to that point, but she now felt a failure for not having been able to give birth naturally and avoided discussions with other mothers because of her sense of shame, so the caesarean was not such a welcome outcome for her later.

Samantha's current obstetrician described feeling 'at sea' in knowing how to help her, and was concerned that she was now requesting an elective caesarean section when there were no obvious medical grounds for this. He suggested that he was not averse to agreeing to this request but needed to understand more about her reasons.

Samantha's presentation at her first appointment with the clinical psychologist was suffused with anger with the maternity staff involved with her previous delivery, and she reported a lack of trust with staff now. She was motivated to have psychological help focused on her previous childbirth experience, but was suspicious of the obstetrician's request for a psychologist's assessment of her reasons for wanting a caesarean, as she was adamant that this was her choice and she did not want a psychologist's report to jeopardise this. Samantha and the clinical psychologist therefore needed to spend some important time at the outset agreeing the psychologist's role and ensuring that all information and decisions were transparent and involved Samantha at all times.

Assessment of Samantha's difficulties was made through clinical interview and use of the Clinical Outcomes in Routine Evaluation (CORE) assessment (Core System Group 1998; a standard measure in the service) and the Impact of Events Scale-Revised (Weiss and Marmar 1996). Her current difficulties included flashbacks to the delivery of her daughter three years earlier whereby she experienced sudden and overwhelming emotions, frightening physical sensations as if re-living the experience, and terrifying images of the birth. She also experienced poor sleep as a direct result of nightmares about the birth, which, on top of the usual tiredness from looking after a young child and being pregnant again, was wearing her down. As mentioned, she was also angry about what she perceived as a lack of care from maternity staff. She was now averse to being examined at all – not just internally – in this pregnancy by the (male) obstetrician (as she had experienced a particularly painful internal examination by a male doctor before), though she had overcome this difficulty with her named midwife by having had time to build a relationship of trust with her. She reported now being phobic of any internal examinations, by any member of staff or her GP, whereas she had previously managed routine smear tests. Samantha was also anxious about going through labour again and felt an elective caesarean was the only option she could consider, even though she felt very upset that she had missed out on a 'normal delivery' and felt shame when talking with other mothers about birth stories. She had a very strong perception of herself as being a 'failure' – as a woman and a mother – for not having been 'successful' with a vaginal delivery and for not being willing to try this again. She had no physical difficulties with her current pregnancy and there were no medical complications. Consultant obstetric involvement for this pregnancy was given because of the previous emergency caesarean and there were uncertain medical grounds at this stage to know whether this would be needed next time. She had no difficulties in her relationship with her three-year old daughter.

The clinical psychologist's intervention with Samantha involved three stages of work. First, it was aimed at reduction or elimination of the most intrusive and disabling traumatic symptoms such as flashbacks. This was conducted by formulating Samantha's difficulties based on a sensorimotor model of trauma (Ogden and Minton 2006), with interventions including Eye Movement Desensitisation and Reprocessing (EMDR). EMDR is an approved therapy for people experiencing post-traumatic stress (NICE 2005), although little used during pregnancy. It is based on the notion that when a person is involved in a distressing event, their brain may afterwards be unable to process the information like a normal memory. In therapy, people are asked to concentrate on images, thoughts and feelings connected to the trauma while at the same time focusing the eyes on something else, such as the therapist's fingers moving from side to side, and being encouraged to let go of the memories and discuss the images and emotions experienced during the eye movements. This serves to stimulate the frozen or blocked information processing system and ultimately allows difficult memories to be replaced by more 'ordinary' memories or positive thoughts. It can be an intense psychological therapy, and is not usually recommended during the first trimester. There is no evidence that there are poor outcomes for the developing foetus, but without more research it is understandable that therapists and pregnant women are wary of intense therapy that can raise adrenaline and cortisol levels. Samantha and the psychologist discussed EMDR and decided against it initially, but Samantha later reconsidered when she weighed up the possible risks of the high levels of stress she was experiencing every day anyway. The outcome of this stage for Samantha was that she experienced massive reduction of all trauma symptoms, with nightmares and flashbacks eliminated and her only becoming moderately upset about the previous delivery when she chose to think about it, rather than having the intrusive unbidden reminders of before.

The second stage involved decision-making about the next delivery, drawing out the pros and cons and considering a 'birth flow diagram' rather than a 'birth plan'. This simple change of language was key in terms of choice and being prepared, but also in helping Samantha to accept that she could not control or predict everything. This stage also, importantly, involved the therapist writing to the obstetrician to give a psychological account of Samantha's difficulties and her decision to ask for an elective caesarean, given Samantha's initial suspicion about a psychologist's role in what is a medical and personal decision. This letter was written in consultation with Samantha and only sent after she gave permission. The decision to ask for a 'planned' caesarean, although having mixed evidence in terms of medicine and research, was a happy outcome for Samantha psychologically; she felt it had helped her 'heal' because it was the most predictable way she could feel in control. The simple change of language from 'elective caesarean' to 'planned caesarean' radically changed Samantha's perception from thinking she would be seen as 'lazy', or 'frivolous', or 'a coward', to thinking that a planned caesarean could be seen as being for valid medical reasons rather than purely personal choice. This stage of work also involved preparation for birth and dealing with procedures and experiences that might remind her of the previous labour and possibly trigger trauma responses.

The final stage of work was a review following the birth of her healthy second child. Samantha's experiences did not lead to any difficulty bonding with the new baby, and she did not experience any re-visiting of the previous trauma. She no longer felt 'less of a mother' because she had not delivered vaginally, so even though it was a second caesarean, this had not increased her feelings of failure. She was now more able to discuss birth stories with other mothers and seemed less concerned about being judged, so she was now more able to use support from others about being a mother. In terms of the future, although a vaginal delivery after two caesarean sections is not likely to be medically indicated, Samantha does not now feel so downcast about 'missing out', but she also hopes that by having not felt traumatised this time around and having experienced more negotiation with maternity staff, she would feel more confident in trusting maternity staff and even to try a vaginal delivery for a third child if that were possible.

Case study 9: Psychological care in the hospice

Mrs Angela Arnold was diagnosed with breast cancer after discovering a breast lump four years ago, at the age of 54. Her treatment included a mastectomy of her affected breast and a course of six cycles of chemotherapy, followed by hormonal tablets, which she has continued to take. Angela was naturally shocked by her initial diagnosis, but felt that she had coped well with the surgery and chemotherapy with support from her husband and grown-up daughter. After a period of 12 months she had returned to her work as a dental receptionist, and apart from occasional feelings of anxiety about her health, particularly around the time of her oncology follow-up appointments, had felt proud at her ability to leave her cancer behind her.

Angela had visited her GP a month ago experiencing back pain. Both she and her GP thought that this was most likely to be related to overdoing her gardening over the summer months, but arranged a precautionary bone scan and appointment with her oncologist. At this appointment her oncologist broke the news to her that she had secondary spread of her disease to her spine. He informed her that metastatic disease could not be cured but that she could be offered calcium treatment to strengthen her bones and further oral chemotherapy with an aim of controlling the disease.

Angela returned to her GP a fortnight later describing high levels of anxiety, periods of weeping and feeling unable to go out of the house. She had not felt able to return to her job as she did not feel able to face her colleagues. She felt that she had let down her family, and that the hospital had failed her by not offering her a bone scan as a routine precaution earlier. She described waking in the night with thoughts about dying, about leaving her daughter and baby grand-daughter. She described feeling very alone and afraid.

Her GP referred her to a palliative care team, based at the local hospice, where she was initially assessed by a clinical nurse specialist in palliative care.

Brennan (2004) notes that cancer recurrence is a devastating time for patients and their families, in which prior hopes of cure are dashed and old feelings from the time of the initial diagnosis may re-emerge. NICE (2004b) Supportive and Palliative care guidelines recommend that the psychological well-being of all patients and carers should be explicitly assessed at key points in the patient's pathway, which includes at the time of recurrence. They also recommend that all staff responsible for patient care should offer patients general emotional support based on skilled communication, effective provision of information, courtesy and respect.

With these guidelines in mind, the clinical nurse specialist visited Angela at home and made an assessment of her holistic needs, which she structured using the Distress Thermometer, a tool which helps to elicit a patient's concern around their physical health, financial, social, emotional and spiritual concerns (Gessler *et al.* 2008). The nurse was also able to offer her some time to reflect on the enormity of the news, to listen to her concerns and to allow her to express her feelings of fear, sadness and anger. She was able to reassure

Angela that her feelings were understandable given the enormity of her experience and that it was the cancer and not her that was the problem.

The nurse was able to work with Angela to develop a plan together, which included a follow-up interview a week later and liaison with the GP to address concerns about the management of her back pain. Angela began to disclose that she had felt alone and lost like this in the past. She described the loss of her mother who had died of breast cancer 10 years previously, and began to talk more about her sadness about the loss of her breast and to experience disturbing memories and flashbacks relating to her mastectomy.

NICE Guidelines (2004b) also recommend that patients and carers found to have significant psychological distress should be offered prompt referral to services able to offer specialist psychological care. The clinical nurse specialist, recognising that Angela's emotional reactions were complicated by other factors which she had not resolved, referred her to a Clinical Health Psychologist working with the palliative care team. The Clinical Health Psychologist made a further assessment of her difficulties, building on the information gathered by the nurse, and she was then able to offer a psychological intervention which focused on reducing Angela's traumatic memories and exploring her sense of loss and uncertainty for the future. Angela and the Clinical Health Psychologist were able to work together to understand how the experience of having lost her mother, her breast and now her sense of loss of a healthy future had intensified her feelings of sadness and anxiety. She was able to express her feelings of grief for her losses within the safe and trusting relationship that developed between the psychologist and herself. The psychologist helped her understand that flashbacks and memories related to the mastectomy were a normal response to such a traumatic experience. Angela was able to describe and process these unwanted thoughts and images so that they became less frequent and less intrusive (Sage *et al.* 2008; Brennan 2004).

The clinical nurse specialist continued to support Angela as she adapted to her new treatment regime and gradually as her anxiety became manageable she felt able to return to part-time work. This return to work was really important to her. She described feeling that it restored some of her sense of her 'old self' and that while things would never be the same again she began to find enjoyment in her friendships, her family and in returning to pottering in her garden.

In this chapter, we have considered elements of psychological care as they might be delivered in a number of health care contexts, and in relation to a number of different patient experiences. In addition, we have considered the more intensive and focused work that may be possible through referral to specialist psychological services, while at the same time bearing in mind the importance of inter-professional working and ongoing liaison with everyone involved in the patients' care. In the final chapter of this book, we consider potential barriers to psychological care delivery and strategies that might begin to address such barriers.

9 The future for psychological care in the twenty-first century

Caring will always be central to nursing, which practises the art of caring using the best of science and technology.

(Nursing and Midwifery Council 2010)

Introduction

With the opening quotation from the NMC, we seem to have come full circle from Chapter 1 in declaring that caring is the core of nursing, and perhaps of other professions too, despite rapid advances in science and technology in the professional health care context. However, within a twenty-first century health care context there are many challenges to providing an optimum service to our patients, particularly in relation to meeting their psychological care needs. In this chapter, we consider the challenges of developing the relevant skills and knowledge to deliver effective psychological care within a modern health care system. Specifically, we explore barriers to effective psychological care within the context of a technically advanced and advancing health care system. Furthermore, we consider potential barriers arising out of a market economy approach to health care provision and within a context of a stringent economy and pressure on health services to 'do more with less'. We consider further the impact on carers when psychological care cannot be delivered effectively, and discuss the concept of 'emotional labour'.

In response to these challenges, we consider what can be done to maintain and improve psychological care skills within a dynamic health care context. We consider the factors involved in learning psychological skills; the relationship between theory and practice; the extent to which education and training can contribute to increasing knowledge; and what an educational curriculum that is psychologically focused might look like. Finally, we consider the role and impact of initiatives such as National Service Frameworks, National Institute for Health and Clinical Excellence (NICE) guidelines, and the Essence of Care strategy and toolkit in alerting practitioners to pay particular focus to the psychological needs of their patients.

Barriers to psychological care delivery

Action point

Assuming that you are convinced of the need to pay attention to your patients' psychological needs, what might prevent you from doing this?

In Chapter 4 we noted that lack of time, competing priorities, an unsupportive clinical environment, and negative attitudes on the part of some staff can stand in the way of delivering psychological care. However, we also noted that psychological care is often delivered most effectively through 'small acts' of caring alongside physical care delivery, and may not add much to the time taken for physical caring (Priest 2010). You may have noted, too, that carers are very rarely specifically trained for a psychological caregiving role, and although implicit within most health care educational curricula, caring per se has not been greatly evident in pre-qualification programmes nor in staff development programmes (Peacock and Nolan 2000). Furthermore, practice guidelines and policies rarely describe explicitly what is meant by psychological care, nor how it can be delivered and evaluated, and there are few easy to use tools readily available to assist in the assessment process.

Later in this chapter we examine a selection of such guidance to explore its contribution to psychological care. Finally, you may have noted that psychological care is not often explicitly documented and as a consequence the effectiveness of any psychological care that is delivered is not often evaluated. We examine some of these barriers, commencing with the culture of the care environment, particularly in relation to technical and technological advances.

External barriers

Care in a technical and technological world

The increased use of technology in health care practice can serve as an actual or perceived barrier to psychological care delivery. Awareness of the existence of such barriers to care, and the consequences of ignoring them, is not a recent development. In her seminal work Watson (1988: 32) stated:

> As the human threats from biotechnology, scientific engineering, fragmented treatment, bureaucracy, and depersonalisation increase and spread in our health care delivery system, so must we increase and spread the human care philosophy, knowledge and practices in our system.

As we noted in Chapter 1, realising that the increase of technology and bureaucracy in nursing had led to an emphasis on curing rather than caring, Watson concluded that it was necessary to restore the balance between cure and care and to view caring as a 'moral imperative'. While it is true that attention to technical equipment places demands on carers' time, there is also the potential for carers to use technology as a barrier in order to avoid the psychosocial aspects of care (Fletcher 1997). The type of care environment in which carrying out physical tasks and paying attention to technological equipment take priority has been described as a 'psychological desert' (Nichols 1993: 192), and staff often experience pressure, in such an environment, to make themselves busy by carrying out practical tasks or engaging in impersonal activities (see Figure 4.3).

Peacock and Nolan (2000) suggest, though, that there is an inherent tension in replacing some caring activities with scientific technologies. While caring should be an expression of humanity, it has been devalued since the mid-nineteenth century in the wake of positivist philosophies. Furthermore, its devaluation has been supported by a National Health Service dominated by illness and cure rather than care. They advocate for a new definition and philosophy of caring, in which scientific and technological approaches supplement caring, and suggest that services based on care may be more cost-effective than those which are not.

In their paper, however, Barnard and Sandelowski (2000) question whether technology and humane care are in fact irreconcilable within contemporary health care environments. They propose that it is not technology (such as medical machinery and equipment) itself that is the problem; rather how such technology is used, and suggest that it is the role of carers to embrace technological advances and thus span the divide between technology and humane health care. This view is endorsed by McGee (2005: 196) who suggests that caring in nursing is 'as much about the type of person the nurse is, how he or she thinks and learns . . . as it is about the ability to use sophisticated technology or employ specialist clinical knowledge'. It is further supported by the NMC (2010: 4) in their lay guidance on pre-registration nursing training, stating that 'care that is competent as well as compassionate is grounded in scientific knowledge and appropriate use of technology as well as in humanitarian professional values'. But there are other challenges facing today's carers, particularly in the light of frequent changes of government policy and changes in what are identified as priority areas for limited resources.

Market economy and economic pressures in the health service

It is widely acknowledged that the development of a freely available and accessible National Health Service in the UK in 1948 was a hugely important innovation, but one that has perhaps become a victim of its own success (McGee 2005), because people are living longer and healthier lives, and are thus placing excessive demands on a health service that continues to be free at the point of delivery. In recent years, successive governments have produced a number of health service reforms aimed at improving efficiency and effectiveness within an increasingly tight budget.

The development of an internal market has dominated UK government policy since the early 1990s (National Archives 1990, Brereton and Vasoodaven 2010). The aims of the internal market were to promote competition and reduce costs, while at the same time increasing efficiency, quality, innovation, and responsiveness. Strategies included separating the functions of care purchasing and care provision via a 'business' model; the development of general practitioner (GP) fund-holding for purchasing care from hospitals; a new responsibility placed upon Regional Health Authorities for purchasing all other health care services; and the creation of self-governing hospital groups (NHS Trusts). Patient choice was to be a key element of the strategy.

While some positive outcomes of these early reforms have been reported, there is limited evidence to support them (Brereton and Vasoodaven 2010), and some evidence that they have not been successful. For example, GP fund-holding was thought to have improved the quality and responsiveness of care provision and achieved reductions in patient waiting times, but may instead have led to various inequities in patient care. Overall, however, the 1990s market policy led to a general increase in patient satisfaction with NHS care and a gradual strengthening of patient choice, both of which should have impacted positively on psychological care.

With a change of government, further reforms took place in 2002 (Department of Health 2002) and these continued to focus on increasing choice for patients, decreasing waiting times, and improving quality of care. This new Act provided for the establishment of Primary Care Trusts and quasi-autonomous Foundation Trusts to purchase and commission community-based and speciality services. It also encouraged purchasers of services to contract with the private and voluntary sector as well as NHS providers, and patients were to be offered a choice of care provider at the time of referral.

Almost before these reforms had had time to be fully evaluated for their impact on patient care, a further change in government introduced new reforms. At the time of writing, further radical changes to the NHS were being proposed as the 2011 Health and Social Care Bill was passing through parliament. This Bill proposes to create an independent NHS Board to allocate resources, promote patient choice, and to reduce NHS administration costs by, for example, abolishing Primary Care Trusts and Strategic Health Authorities, almost before they have had time to establish themselves and to provide stability for carers and patients alike in their experience of the health care system.

Gordon (1991 cited in Staden 1998) was critical of the 'invasion of the marketplace into the caring professions' and feared that converting a human service into a commodity would result in cut-backs and an emphasis on efficiency at the expense of individualised and personalised care. Overall, it is likely that factors arising out of a market-orientated approach to care delivery within the NHS such as managerialism and a performance culture have resulted in an over-riding concern with the achievement of targets, cost-effectiveness and financial stringency. One of the effects of this is rapid in-patient turnover, coupled with an expansion in the range of procedures undertaken on a day patient basis or within General Practitioner surgeries, potentially resulting in staff being unable to know their patients well enough to identify their psychological care needs. In relation to the current reforms, the Royal College of Nursing (2011) has expressed concerns about the large scale and rapid pace of change. Specifically, the College is concerned that recent improvements in patient care (including decreased waiting times, better outcomes, improved access and flexibility of services, as well as more clinical staff) would be jeopardised; that there could be variations in service; and that there could be reduced collaboration and sharing of good practice, all of which could have an adverse impact on the quality of care delivery.

At the time of writing, the English government had recently conducted a comprehensive spending review and required the NHS to save £20 billion over the next four years. It is difficult to envisage how such stringent cuts could fail to impact on patient care, and to result in psychological care being delivered as an add-on or luxury part of care delivery, as feared by Nichols as long ago as 1993.

Internal barriers

Having considered some potential external constraints on psychological care delivery in the twenty-first century, we turn our attention now to internal barriers, focusing specifically on how carers manage the stress of caring and protect themselves from any ensuing anxiety. We consider the concepts of defence from anxiety and emotional labour, and consider whether these are valid and current barriers to psychological care delivery today.

As long ago as 1960, Isabel Menzies Lyth wrote about the importance of understanding nursing within the context of the environment in which it was practiced (her observations at the time were conducted within hospital settings). She conceptualised the hospital as a social system which was likely to create anxiety amongst its employees in the caring professions, given the physically and emotionally demanding nature of the work. She argued that carers tended to defend themselves against this anxiety by 'establishing protective shells, projecting negative attitudes or . . . defensive behaviour' (Ross 2010). Menzies Lyth observed that nurses preferred to be task oriented to protect them from dealing with the suffering of others.

Developing this theme, James (1992), and Smith and Gray (2001) explored the concept and effects of 'emotional labour' as a way of managing the stress of caring. The term was first coined by Hochschild in 1983 in relation to professional groups providing services, such as airline stewards and debt collectors, but it has subsequently been applied widely to the caring professions. Emotional labour can be defined as 'the management of feeling' or 'the induction or suppression of feeling in order to sustain the outward appearance that produces the proper state of mind in others – that of being cared for in a safe and a convivial place' (cited in Staden 1998: 149). It describes what happens when there is a mis-match between the actual emotions experienced by a carer and the emotions that carers feel they *ought* to experience. What happens then is a form of 'emotion work' where the carer tries to convey or act what they feel is the appropriate emotion. For example, a carer might say to him or herself: 'I feel angry with that patient who is not motivated to do her mobilisation exercises, but I ought to empathise with her because she feels low and has low self esteem'. Managing the expression of emotion is demanding and the consequences, ultimately, can be worker alienation, burnout (sometimes referred to as compassion fatigue), stress, and low professional performance (Cropanzano, Weiss and Elias 2003). Furthermore, students and junior staff are likely to model their own management of conflicting emotions by observing the strategies of more senior colleagues, and thus encourage the spread of emotional labour within the workplace.

The need for staff support to counteract the burden of caring has been well identified within the literature (e.g. Nichols 1993), but the findings of Priest's (2001) study suggested that formal systems of staff support and clinical supervision are not widely available. However, the study revealed some of the lengths to which nurses will go to ensure that they are able to access support for their psychological caregiving role, such as consulting external experts, forming informal support groups, or seeking informal supervisory relationships with colleagues. While long recognised as an important element of mental health nursing practice, clinical psychology, social work and counselling, the widespread adoption of clinical supervision in general nursing settings has been slower, although its implementation is gathering momentum (Heath and Freshwater 2000). It has been established that clinical supervision has a beneficial impact on staff, and, where it has not been introduced, measurable detrimental effects (Butterworth *et al.* 1997). The implication is that without appropriate supervision, nurses' reflective abilities will be reduced (see Chapter 5), and this will in turn hamper the provision of psychological care. Furthermore, participation in clinical supervision is recognised as a way of exercising clinical responsibility. The lack of formal supervision led nurses in Priest's study either to seek out their own sources of supervision and support, or not to receive them at all. We have considered in previous chapters the potentially negative consequences for both patients and carers of not providing psychological care. In the current stringent emotional climate it is easy to envisage that staff support mechanisms, where they exist, are likely to assume low priority, with a potential knock on effect on staff stress, emotional labour, and burnout and ultimately on the quality of care delivery.

With these internal and external barriers acknowledged, what strategies are at our disposal in the modern health care environment to enhance the profile of psychological health care delivery? We move on now to consider the role and challenges of education in promoting and enhancing the centrality of psychological care within a challenging contemporary health care environment.

Learning to care

In Chapters 5, 6 and 7 we outlined the requisite personal qualities, skills and knowledge underpinning effective psychological care delivery. But how do health care professionals learn to care, and in particular, to deliver psychological care? How well does theoretical learning translate into skilled practice? We shall, as in other chapters, consider these opportunities in relation to nursing and nursing education; however similar issues are likely to be relevant across other health care preparation programmes.

As long ago as 1979, Rimon suggested that nurses were 'not being provided with the necessary knowledge of the psychological, cultural and social components of health and illness'. This view continued to be endorsed 15 years later: 'Although staff members generally support the need for psychological interventions, they often do not have the confidence, skill or power to alter perceived priorities and traditions in caring for patients' (Wilson-Barnett 1994b: 26), and it is still recognised that nurses require training, assistance and support to function effectively in this area (Priest 1999a).

Even when nurses have received training and support, they are likely still to feel uncertain about how to intervene (Barry 1996). Court (1995) pointed out that nursing staff have often received inadequate training to pay sufficient attention to the psychological aspects of patient care, and that their efforts to do so are not encouraged in practice. Bennett (1994) expressed disappointment that, as a consequence, the skills and strategies for psychological caregiving were available to so few patients.

Translating theory into practice

In this book we have considered aspects of psychological knowledge and skill that might help us in developing psychological care. But what evidence is there that health care professionals do in fact translate scientific knowledge and theory into practical hands on care? Many writers have indentified the theory–practice gap, pointing out that is it difficult to provide evidence for a direct relationship between knowledge and care delivery.

It is clear from an examination of nursing curricula and educational texts that psychological knowledge has, over the years, had some influence upon nursing education and practice. As we saw in Chapter 2, the precise nature of this influence has varied according to the beliefs and practices dominant in psychology at the time. It is true that some of the most obvious applications (for example, psychotherapeutic approaches, behaviour therapy and modification, group therapeutic approaches and cognitive therapy) have been most evident in mental health and intellectual disability contexts, rather than in general adult nursing settings. Nonetheless, psychological knowledge has made its mark in nursing generally through the widespread acceptance of, for example, counselling skills as part of nursing's repertoire, and continues to make an impact through the growing field of health psychology. However, despite the efforts of many writers and researchers to stress the relationship between psychological knowledge and psychological care, there is little evidence that nurses themselves make the link, and although we have offered some suggestions in Chapter 7, it remains unclear exactly what range and type of knowledge would best facilitate the forging of this link and the delivery of the best possible care. Thus, despite the long acknowledged association between nursing and psychology, and considerable interest in the ways in which psychological concepts have been applied in practice, psychology seems not to have had a major impact upon the teaching of nurses and other health care professionals. Furthermore, it has somehow failed to affect practice, being seen as the province of writers, academics, and to some extent, teachers of nursing.

Findings from Priest's (2001, 2006) study would support this. Student and qualified nurses were asked about how they expected to acquire, or had acquired, psychological caregiving abilities. Most believed that a core of the required abilities was implicit within pre-existing personal qualities. In other words, some people would naturally be good at psychological caregiving, while others would not.

However, they thought that these pre-existing qualities could be enhanced and developed through experiences in practice; through observing and imitating the behaviours of key role models, and through reflecting upon their own actions and interactions (Priest 2006).

Unfortunately, neither students nor qualified nurses believed that formal education programmes played much more than a peripheral role in the acquisition of psychological caregiving abilities.

There seems, then, to be a need to introduce strategies into educational programmes that will promote psychological caregiving as an integral part of everyday holistic care.

Specifically, we need to enhance carers' ability to 'recognise psychological needs, understand the factors that influence individual psychological responses, and to respond appropriately to these individual expressions of need and responses' (Priest 2006).

Unfortunately, there is little available research evidence about the nature and effectiveness of psychological care education programmes, and clearly, no preparatory or continuing education programme can address barriers to care delivery arising out of the market economy or stringent financial constraint. Furthermore, costly continuing professional education programmes are themselves likely to be a victim of financial pressures and cutbacks. Nonetheless, professional health care preparation programmes can provide an opportunity to enhance the status of care and psychological care. With that in mind, the challenge then is to design relevant educational strategies to enhance psychological care delivery, within the context of contemporary health care programmes developed according to statutory guidelines (e.g. NMC 2010).

Over the years, several solutions have been proposed in an attempt to make psychological knowledge more accessible and relevant within nursing curricula. Girot (1991), for example, advocated social psychology as a medium through which academic knowledge from psychology and sociology could be meaningfully linked. In contrast, Chapman and Fields (1992) advocated that humanistic psychology, and in particular, counselling, should be the basis of the curriculum. In this way, interpersonal and therapeutic skills would be integrated as core themes. Suggested content in such a curriculum would focus on the skills required by nurses to orientate to clients' needs, to listen, offer free attention, suspend preconception, offer empathy, feel and show acceptance, respect and warmth, and help patients with their coping strategies. As well as having positive outcomes for patients, such a basis to the curriculum should also improve students' self-esteem and confidence, and ensure interpersonal support. However, it is clear that such a curriculum would rely heavily upon suitably experienced and confident teachers.

Morrison and Burnard (1997b) produced practical guidance for nurse educators in the form of a facilitator's manual to accompany their text on caring and communicating, in which psychological care is a major component. Morrison (1993) also considered the teaching strategies required to facilitate the integration and application of psychological knowledge. Following a review of the teaching content and methods used in Australian universities he concluded that problem-based learning (PBL) was an appropriate approach. Popular within medical curricula in the UK for some time, the PBL approach is beginning to impact upon nursing and other health care curricula, and, if thoroughly exploited as a teaching and learning strategy, should ensure that all the appropriate knowledge and skill relevant to a particular patient problem is obtained and considered. However, this strategy assumes adequate preparation and skill on the part of educators acting as PBL facilitators to ensure comprehensive coverage, and there is scope for emphasising or minimising the importance of certain aspects of the selected problem in accordance with their own knowledge, experience, expertise or orientation. There are many other accounts and reviews of training programmes designed to improve elements of psychological care delivery in specific contexts, such as oncology (e.g. Sheldon 2007), with most claiming improvement in communication skills and confidence and some evidence of these improvements lasting over time.

Arising out of Priest's (2001, 2006) research, a framework and content for the psychological care strand of the curriculum was produced, aiming to give a higher profile to the concept of psychological care, to emphasise skills development underpinned by personal and professional development strategies, and to encompass relevant psychological knowledge, from which to understand individual reactions.

Within such a programme, teaching and learning strategies are essentially experiential and might include:

Skills development activities

For example:

- counselling skills exercises
- case-based and problem based learning
- role play and feedback
- video and audio recorded work with feedback
- use of simulated environments and simulated patients (as is common in medical education)

Personal and professional development activities

For example:

- *self awareness* – games, feedback, positive reinforcement
- *self care* – stress management skills, relaxation training, group work
- *assertiveness skills*

(Priest 2006)

Students and educators alike often evaluate such activities positively, particularly the opportunity to work in small cohesive groups with continuity of educator input; the availability of educators and other students as role models; the opportunity to take risks, to self disclose, and obtain feedback in a safe environment; and the opportunity to reflect on personal development and areas of difficulty. Within a tightly packed curriculum, however, time would need to be found to support learning in this labour intensive way alongside learning factual knowledge and practical and clinical skills. A further challenge is to adapt what are essentially small group activities for potentially large groups of students (Burnard 1993b, Priest 2006). Furthermore, such activities are costly both in terms of human and material resources (such as rooms and equipment) and the emotional demands placed on students and educators.

Despite these challenges and costs, it is hoped that such investment would enhance the development of carers' psychological caregiving abilities, to the ultimate benefit of their patients (Priest 2006).

Current educational guidance

Skills based and personal development activities are not incompatible with recent guidance on the content and delivery of undergraduate health care programmes, such as the Nursing and Midwifery Council (NMC 2007) guidance on simulated learning. This guidance on using simulated learning environments as part of students' practical experience allows an opportunity for them to practise skills, including psychological care skills, in a realistic but safe environment and to obtain feedback on their emerging skills. Evaluation of such simulation opportunities suggests that this is an effective way of supporting learning.

Key principles of psychological care are implicit within the NMC (2010) guidance on pre-registration education in the UK, although it does not specifically detail the learning strategies needed to develop such skills. As well as heralding an all-graduate entry route into the profession of nursing, this guidance is derived from what the public has said it wants from nurses when they come into a health care context. The public wants nurses to be effective communicators, demonstrating compassion and integrity, and skilled at sharing decisions about care appropriately. The public also wants nurses who understand that people's back-grounds, environments and ways of life might influence their health, and who recognise the impact that different care contexts might have upon people's unique personalities and situations. In response, the NMC guidance identifies five essential skills clusters to be incorporated into all pre-registration educational programmes, the first two of which are care, compassion and communication; and organisational aspects of care. Although the skills clusters do not make specific reference to 'psychological care', there is regular and clear signposting to the elements of holistic care, for example, at the point of entry to the professional nursing register. After three years of preparation, nurses should (amongst many other skills) be able to make 'a holistic, person-centred and systematic assessment of physical, emotional, psychological, social, cultural and spiritual needs'. Other implicit evidence can be seen in requirements for nurses to engage with people and build caring professional relationships, use professional support structures, be self aware and confident yet know their limitations, act as role models, take a person-centred personalised approach to care, and act professionally to ensure judgements, prejudices, values, attitudes and beliefs do not compromise care. More specific skills include listening to, watching for, and respond-ing to non-verbal cues, and using the skills of active listening, questioning, paraphrasing and reflection, all of which we have seen are essential ingredients of counselling skills, which are in turn necessary in psychological care delivery.

Having considered how educational strategies can enhance the prominence of psycho-logical care within the modern twenty-first century health care environment, we turn now to examples of practice strategies and guidelines that might help to focus carers' minds on the centrality of psychological elements of care. We consider National Service Frameworks (NSFs), the role of the National Institute for Health and Clinical Effectiveness (NICE) and its guidance, and the Essence of Care Strategy, in a number of examples of clinical practice.

National Service Frameworks

National Service Frameworks (NSFs) are long-term strategies for improving specific areas of care. They set national standards for care and measurable goals 'based on the best available evidence of what treatments and services work most effectively for patients' (NHS Choices 2010). There are NSFs in existence for the following health conditions: cancer (we have already discussed the NHS Cancer Reform strategy, 2007, which is the current NSF for cancer, in Chapter 8), chronic obstructive pulmonary disease (COPD), coronary heart disease, stroke, diabetes, and long-term conditions, and in relation to the following services: mental health, older people, children and maternity, and renal services.

Action point

Identify and access the NSF that is most relevant to your area of practice, using the Department of Health website (www.dh.org.uk). Identify any elements of the framework that you think could support you in delivering effective psychological care.

Space precludes a detailed discussion of specific frameworks here, but as an example, we will examine the NSF for coronary heart disease. This framework includes a chapter on cardiac rehabilitation (defined in the NSF as 'activities required to influence favourably the underlying cause of the disease, as well as the best possible, physical, mental and social conditions, so that . . . [patients] may . . . preserve or resume . . . as normal a place as possible in the community'). In this chapter of the framework recommendations are made that before discharge from hospital, patients who have had a myocardial infarction (heart attack) or other cardiac event are offered a full assessment of their physical, psychological and social needs and that an individual plan is negotiated for each patient detailing these needs in writing, to be shared between the patient and the GP. It is recommended that advice is given on lifestyle activities including sexual activity and employment, and that patients are given information about cardiac support groups and other locally relevant information.

In this way, it is fully acknowledged that a serious cardiac event will impact on all areas of a patient's functioning. Information needs are fully acknowledged, as emphasised in Chapter 6, as is the need for ongoing psychosocial support. Thus, a nurse, physiotherapist, occupational therapist, dietician or other professional involved in cardiac rehabilitation can draw on explicit guidelines to help them to prepare the patient for discharge, ensuring that psychological needs are identified and individual plans made to address them.

National Institute for Health and Clinical Effectiveness (NICE) guidelines

NICE is 'an independent organisation responsible for providing national guidance on promoting good health and preventing and treating ill health' within the NHS in England (NICE 2011). Implementing NICE guidance helps to ensure that people have equal access to health care and that consistent improvements are made to the health of the population. An implementation programme has been created to facilitate this. Evidence about the best assessment, treatment and care strategies and the services needed to provide them are readily available for a large number of health problems via the internet. These include cancer, cardiovascular, respiratory, and musculoskeletal problems, together with injuries and accidents and many other physical and mental health conditions, and all have their own list of sub-topics. For example, a sub-topic of the cancer guideline is breast cancer.

Exploring the breast cancer guidelines as an example, we note a section relating to psychosocial support. This section provides evidence that 'on-going contact with a trained and experienced breast care nurse can reduce patients' anxiety, depression and physical symptoms up to a year after treatment' (NICE 2002: 30) and that more formal psychological interventions such as CBT, relaxation therapy, and counselling can reduce psychological disturbances and improve quality of life.

Moving on to examine the guidelines for people with acute onset chest pain (NICE 2010), there is clear recognition that this will be a time of heightened anxiety for the patient and family, and considerable emphasis is placed upon providing information. As part of the extensive guidance on information giving, carers are reminded to take into account the anxiety likely to be experienced when the cause of the chest pain is unknown, to offer a clear explanation of the possible causes of their symptoms and the uncertainties, to correct any misinformation, to provide repeated opportunities for discussion, and to encourage people to ask questions, all key elements of sound psychological care.

Action point

Find NICE guidelines relevant to your own area of clinical practice (see NICE 2011 http://www.nice.org.uk/). How well do these guidelines help you to think about your patients' psychological needs and care? Are the key elements of psychological care delivery to be found within these guidelines? Is anything missing?

Essence of Care strategy

Finally, we consider the contribution of the Essence of Care strategy to enhancing psychological care. Both the national nursing strategy for England, *Making a Difference* (Department of Health 1999) and The NHS Plan (Department of Health 2000) stressed the importance of getting the basics right in terms of care delivery and improving patients' experience of care. As a result, in 2001, the English government introduced the Essence of Care strategy and toolkit, which has since been updated several times; its current version is designed to meet the needs of a range of professionals working in a variety of care settings (Department of Health 2010a). The importance of providing and monitoring high-quality care is seen as central to the provision of health and social care services in the twenty-first century, and the Essence of Care strategy can be used as a tool for sharing and comparing practice, for developing action plans for improvement, and for identifying staff education and training needs. As such, it serves as the national benchmarking system for health and social care. Benchmarking is a means of identifying examples of best practice in care delivery, and using these examples as standards against which to compare actual practice. In this way, it is possible to identify when, and by how much, actual care delivery practices are falling short of the stated benchmark or standard, and to put action plans in place to ensure that the standards can be met. In developing the benchmarks, patients, carers and health care professionals worked together to agree and describe good quality care and best practice.

The Essence of Care strategy focuses on many of the 'softer' aspects of care, which are sometimes difficult to measure objectively, such as ensuring privacy and dignity for patients, and helps professionals to consider these in a structured way. By helping to identify best practice, through sharing and comparing, and remedying poor practice, health care staff can be helped to address issues of concern within their local workplace and make improvements. Currently, twelve areas of care have been identified for the development of benchmarks following a consultation exercise in 2009:

- bladder, bowel and continence care
- care environment
- communication
- food and drink
- prevention and management of pain
- personal hygiene
- prevention and management of pressure ulcers
- promoting health and well-being
- record keeping
- respect and dignity
- safety
- self care

Reflection point

Which of these twelve areas of care do you think are relevant to psychological care delivery, and why?

At first glance, perhaps the most obviously relevant are 'communication', 'respect and dignity' and 'care environment', and we have in previous chapters discussed the centrality of communication skills and the impact of the care environment in promoting, or otherwise, effective psychological care. Thus it is pleasing that these areas are emphasised as areas for developing high quality care. Interestingly, the Royal College of Nursing (2008) has identified communication and respect and dignity as two of the three top priority topics for a national audit of the strategy. Some of the benchmarks, such as 'bladder, bowel and continence care', 'personal and oral hygiene', and 'prevention and management of pressure ulcers' may appear to be much more instrumental or task based in their care focus. However, it should be noted that many of the benchmarks overlap and that it would, for instance, be important to take into account patients' privacy and dignity while attending to bladder or bowel care. Equally, it is difficult to envisage how any area of direct care can be carried out effectively without excellent communication skills.

Therefore, for the purposes of this chapter we will restrict our exploration of 'Essence of Care' to the benchmark for communication, and consider how it can help us to understand, identify and respond to patients' psychological needs. (It should be noted that Essence of Care does not use the term 'patient', referring instead to 'people', but for consistency we continue to use the term patient here.) This benchmark includes a number of general principles as well as specific guidance. General principles include the aim that care should be delivered 'with compassion and empathy in a respectful and non-judgemental way', directly supporting the need for such personal qualities as identified in Chapter 6. A further general principle is maintaining patients' confidentiality and obtaining consent before any intervention is carried out, including sharing information, taking into account individual capacity to consent. Patient choice in developing personalised plans of care is emphasised and there is a requirement that care staff are competent to 'assess, plan, implement, evaluate and revise care according to patients' individual needs'. There is a requirement that all documentation pertaining to patient care is maintained in such a way that it can be available for external scrutiny, and that care is integrated 'with clear and effective communication between . . . staff, people [i.e. patients] and carers'. This is important guidance in relation to documenting the care that is provided beyond physical care, and in relation to referring on and liaising with other professionals as illustrated in Chapter 8.

As well as this general guidance, specific best practice outcomes in relation to communication are documented and include a requirement that all staff demonstrate effective interpersonal skills; that communication takes place at appropriate times and in appropriate environments, that patients' communication needs are assessed and monitored; that information sharing is promoted, and that staff and patients are continuously supported throughout care delivery. These outcomes are all compatible with key elements of psychological care discussed throughout this book (interpersonal skills, assessment and monitoring, informational care, consideration of the care environment, making time for care, and the provision of staff support). Thus the Essence of Care strategy can be seen as a helpful guide in providing competent and effective psychological care.

Conclusion

In this chapter we have considered a number of internal and external constraints that could impact adversely upon the provision of psychological care. It is acknowledged that some of the strategies we have considered for addressing these constraints are 'top–down' and subject to change as new scientific knowledge is developed and new evidence about best practice is identified and verified. However it is clear that in the twenty-first century health and social care environment, considerable emphasis is being placed upon identifying and addressing not just physical needs in illness but also on wider holistic health care needs. Perhaps we can conclude by citing the view of Bor, Gill, Miller and Evans (2009: 43) that while challenges will always arise, 'to ignore the psychological care of the patient is no longer an option in the modern, accountable health care setting'.

References

Aggleton, P. and Chalmers, H. (2000). *Nursing Models and Nursing Practice* (2nd edn). Basingstoke: Macmillan.

Ainsworth, M. and Bell, S. (1970). Attachment, exploration and separation: illustrated by the behaviour of one-year-olds in a strange situation. *Child Development*, 41, pp. 49–65.

Alladdin, W. (2009). An ethnobiopsychosocial human rights model for educating community counsellors globally. *Counselling Psychology Quarterly*, 22(1), pp. 17–24.

Altschul, A. (1962). *Psychology for Nurses*. London: Ballière Tindall and Cassell.

American Holistic Nurses' Association (AHNA) (2010). What is holistic nursing? www.ahna.org/ AboutUs/ WhatisHolisticNursing.

American Psychiatric Association (2000). *Diagnostic and Statistical Manual of Mental Disorders, Text Revision (DSM-IV-TR)*. Philadelphia: APA.

Argyle, M. (1988). *Bodily Communication* (2nd edn). New York: Methuen.

Arnold, E. (1999). Structuring the relationship. In E. Arnold and K. Boggs (Eds), *Interpersonal Relationships. Professional Communication Skills For Nurses* (pp. 80–106). Philadephia: W.B. Saunders Co.

Arthur, A. R. (2003). The emotional lives of people with learning disability. *British Journal of Learning Disabilities*, 31, pp. 25–30.

Asch, S. E. (1946). Forming impressions of personality. *Journal of Abnormal and Social Psychology*, 41, pp. 258–290.

Attree, M. (2001). Patients' and relatives' experiences and perspectives of 'Good' and 'Not so Good' quality care. *Journal of Advanced Nursing*, 33(4), pp. 456–466.

Bach, S. (1995). *Psychology in Practice*. London: South Bank University Distance Learning Centre.

Bach, S. and Grant, A. (2009). *Communication and Interpersonal Skills for Nurses*. Exeter: Learning Matters.

British Association for Counselling and Psychotherapy (BACP) (2010). What is counselling? http://www.bacp.co.uk/information/education/whatiscounselling.php.

Bandura, A. (1989). Perceived self-efficacy in the exercise of personal agency. *The Psychologist*, 10, pp. 411–424.

Barker, P. (Ed.) (2003). *Psychiatric and Mental Health Nursing: The Craft of Caring*. London: Arnold.

Barnard, A. and Sandelowski, M. (2000). Technology and humane nursing care: (ir)reconcilable or invented difference. *Journal of Advanced Nursing*, 34(3), pp. 356–366.

Bauer, J. A. (1990). Caring as the central focus in nursing curriculum development. In M. Leininger and J. Watson (Eds), *The Caring Imperative in Education* (pp. 255–266). New York: National League for Nursing.

Baughan, J. and Smith, A. (2008). *Caring in Nursing Practice*. Harlow: Pearson Education.

Beck, A. T. (1979). *Cognitive Therapy and the Emotional Disorders*. New York: Plume Books.

Beck, A. T., Ward, C. H., Mendelson, M., Mock, J. and Erbaugh, J. (1961). An inventory for measuring depression. *Archives of General Psychiatry*, 4, pp. 561–571.

Beck, C. (1999). Quantitative measurement of caring. *Journal of Advanced Nursing*, 30(1), pp. 24–32.

Bellani, M. L. (2008). Psychological aspects in day-case surgery. *International Journal of Surgery*, 6, Suppl. 1, pp. S44–S46.

Benner, P. (1984). *From Novice to Expert. Excellence and Power in Clinical Nursing Practice*. Menlo Park: Addison-Wesley.

Benner, P. and Tanner, C. (1987). How expert nurses use intuition. *American Journal of Nursing*, 87(1), pp. 23–31.

Benner, P. and Wrubel, J. (1989). *The Primacy of Caring. Stress and Coping in Health and Illne*ss. Menlo Park: Addison-Wesley.

Bennett, P. (1994). Psychological care of the coronary patient. *Journal of Mental Health*, 3(4), pp. 477–484.

Biley, F. (2005). Invisible knowledge. *Nursing Standard*, 19(23), pp. 17–18.

Bishop, A. and Scudder, J. (1991). *Nursing. The Practice of Caring*. New York: National League for Nursing.

Boore, J. (1978). *A Prescription for Recovery*. London: Royal College of Nursing.

Bor, R., Gill, S., Miller, R. and Evans, A. (2009). *Counselling in Health Care Settings*. Basingstoke: Palgrave Macmillan.

Bowlby, J. (1969). *Attachment*. Vol. I. Attachment and Loss. London: Pimlico.

Boykin, A. and Schoenhofer, S. (1993) *Nursing as Caring: A Model For Transforming Practice*. New York: National League for Nursing.

BPS (British Psychological Society) (2010). What do psychologists do? http://www.bps.org.uk/careers/what-do-psychologists-do.

Brechin, A. (1999). What makes for good care? In A. Brechin, J. Walmsley, J. Katz and A. Peace (Eds), *Care Matters* (pp. 170–187). London: Sage.

Brennan, J. (2004). *Cancer in Context: A Practical Guide to Supportive and Palliative Care*. Oxford: Oxford University Press.

Brennan, K. A., Clark, C. L. and Shaver, P. R. (1998). Self-report measurement of adult romantic attachment: an integrative overview. In J. A. Simpson and W. S. Rholes (Eds), *Attachment Theory and Close Relationships* (pp. 46–76). New York: Guilford Press.

Brereton, L. and Vasoodaven, V. (2010). The impact of the NHS market. http://www.civitas.org.uk/nhs/download/Civitas_LiteratureReview_NHS_market_Feb10.pdf.

Bridges, J. (1990). Literature review on the images of the nurse and nursing in the media. *Journal of Advanced Nursing*, 15(7), pp. 850–854.

Bright, M. (1997). Comment. *The Independent*, 28 September, p. 26.

British Holistic Medical Association (2010). http://www.bhma.org/.

Brooker, D. (2004). What is person-centred care for people with dementia? *Reviews in Clinical Gerontology*, 13, pp. 215–222.

Brooker, D. (2005). Dementia care mapping: a review of the research literature. *The Gerontologist 45*, Special Issue I, pp. 11–18.

Brown, J. M., Kitson, A. L. and McKnight, T. J. (1992). *Challenges in Caring. Explorations in Nursing and Ethics*. London: Chapman and Hall.

Brown, L. (1986). The experience of care: patient perspectives. *Topics in Clinical Nursing*, 8(2), pp. 56–62.

Burnard, P. (1993). Using experiential learning methods with large groups of students. *Nurse Education Today*, 13, pp. 60–65.

Burnard, P. (1994a). Analysing data using a wordprocessor. *Nurse Researcher*, 1(3), pp. 33–42.

Burnard, P. (1994b). Searching for meaning: a method of analysing interview transcripts with a personal computer. *Nurse Education Today*, 14, pp. 111–117.

Burnard, P. (1998). Personal qualities or skills? A report of a study of nursing students' views of the characteristics of counsellors. *Nurse Education Today*, 18, pp. 649–654.

Burnard, P. (2005). *Counselling Skills for Health Professionals* (4th edn). Cheltenham: Nelson Thornes.

Carers UK (2007). About us. http://www.carersuk.org/Aboutus.

Carkhuff, R. R. (1969). *Helping and Human Relations: A Primer for Lay and Professional Helpers.* New York: Holt, Rinehart and Winston.

Chapman, T. and Fields, H. (1992). Interpersonal and therapeutic skills in the 'New Curriculum' for nurse education. In K. Soothill, C. Henry and K. Kendrick (Eds), *Themes and Perspectives in Nursing* (pp. 101–113). London: Chapman and Hall.

Chipman, Y. (1991). Caring: its meaning and place in the practice of nursing. *Journal of Nursing Education*, 30(4), pp. 171–175.

Clarke, J. and Wheeler, S. (1992). A view of the phenomenon of caring in nursing practice. *Journal of Advanced Nursing*, 17(11), pp. 1283–1290.

Clifford, C. (1995). Caring: fitting the concept to nursing practice. *Journal of Clinical Nursing*, 4, pp. 37–41.

Colaizzi, P. F. (1978). Psychological research as the phenomenologist views it. In R. Valle and M. King (Eds), *Existential-Phenomenological Alternatives for Psychology* (pp. 48–71). New York: Oxford Press.

Core System Group (1998). *CORE System (Information Management) Handbook.* Leeds: Core System Group.

Cropanzano, R., Weiss, H. and Elias, S. (2003). The impact of display rules and emotional labor on psychological well-being at work. In P. Perrewé and D. Ganster (Eds), *Emotional and Physiological Processes and Positive Intervention Strategies (Research in Occupational Stress and Well-being, Volume 3)* (pp. 45–89). Bingley: Emerald Group Publishing Limited.

Cutcliffe, J. and Cassedy, P. (1999). The development of empathy in students on a short, skills based counselling course: a pilot study. *Nurse Education Today*, 19, pp. 250–257.

Danziger, K. (1990). *Constructing the Subject. Historical Origins of Psychological Research.* Cambridge: Cambridge University Press.

Danziger, K. (1997). *Naming the Mind. How Psychology found its Language.* London: Sage.

Davies, C. (1999). Caregiving, carework and professional care. In A. Brechin, J. Walmsley, J. Katz and A. Peace, *Care Matters* (pp. 126–138). London: Sage.

Davis, B. (2000). *Caring for People in Pain.* London: Routledge.

Davis, H. and Fallowfield, L. (Eds) (1991). *Counselling and Communication in Health Care.* Chichester: Wiley.

Davis, T. M., Maguire, T. O., Haraphongse, M. and Schaumberger, M. R. (1994). Preparing patients for cardiac catheterisation: informational treatment and coping interactions. *Heart & Lung*, 23, pp. 130–139.

Denscombe, M. (1998). *The Good Research Guide.* Buckingham: Open University Press.

Department of Health (1999). *Making a Difference. Strengthening the Nursing, Midwifery, and Health Visiting Contribution to Health and Healthcare.* London: Department of Health.

Department of Health (2000). *The NHS Plan: A Plan for Investment, A Plan for Reform.* London: Department of Health.

Department of Health (2002). NHS Reform and Health Care Professions Act. http://www.dh.gov.uk/en/ Publicationsandstatistics/Legislation/Actsandbills/DH_4002186.

Department of Health (2009). *Living Well with Dementia: A National Dementia Strategy.* London: Department of Health.

Department of Health (2010a). *Essence of Care 2010.* London: The Stationery Office. http://www.dh. gov.uk/prod_consum_dh/groups/dh_digitalassets/@dh/@en/@ps/documents/digitalasset/dh_11 9978.pdf.

Department of Health (2010b). Quality outcomes for people with dementia: building on the work of the National Dementia Strategy. http://www.dh.gov.uk/en/Publicationsandstatistics/Publications/ PublicationsPolicyAndGuidance/DH_119827.

Department of Health (2011). Health and Social Care Bill. http://www.publications.parliament.uk/pa/ cm201011/cmbills/132/11132.i–v.html#top.

de Raeve, L. (2010). Passing on the blame. In L. de Raeve, M. Rafferty and M. Paget, *Nurses and Their Patients: Informing Practice Through Psychodynamic Insights* (pp. 57–72). Keswick: M&K Publishing.

Devine, E. C. (1992). Effects of psycho-educational care for adult surgical patients: a meta-analysis of 191 studies. *Patient Education and Counselling*, 19, pp. 129–142.

Di Blasi, Z., Harkness, E., Ernst, E., Georgiou, A. and Kleijnen, J. (2001). Influence of context effects on health outcomes: a systematic review. *The Lancet*, 357, pp. 757–762.

Diekelmann, N. (1993). Transforming RN education: new approaches to innovation. *National League for Nursing Publications, 14–2511*, pp. 42–57.

Doka, K. J. (1989). *Disenfranchised Grief: Recognizing Hidden Sorrow*. Toronto, Canada: Lexington Books.

Egan, G. (2001). *The Skilled Helper: A Problem-Management and Opportunity-Development Approach to Helping* (7th edn). Stamford: Wadsworth.

Ekman, P. (2004). *Emotions Revealed: Understanding Faces and Feelings*. London: Phoenix.

Ersser, S. (1990). A search for the therapeutic dimensions of nurse–patient interaction. In R. McMahon and A. Pearson (Eds), *Nursing as Therapy* (pp. 43–84). London: Chapman and Hall.

Eysenck, M. (2009). *Fundamentals of Psychology*. Hove: Psychology Press.

Farrell, G. A. (1991). How accurately do nurses perceive patients' needs? A comparison of general and psychiatric settings. *Journal of Advanced Nursing*, 16, pp. 1062–1070.

Federoff, H. J. and Gostin, L. O. (2009). Evolving from reductionism to holism: is there a future for systems medicine? *Journal of the American Medical Association* 302, 9, pp. 994–996.

Feil, N. (1991). Validation therapy. In P. Kim, *Serving the Elderly: Skills for Practice* (pp. 89–115). Piscataway, NJ: Transaction Publishers.

Fisher, B. and Tronto, J. (1990). Toward a feminist theory of care. In E. Abel and M. Nelson (Eds), *Circles of Care: Work and Identity in Women's Lives* (pp. 34–62). Albany, NY: State University of New York Press.

Fletcher, J. (1997). Do nurses really care? Some unwelcome findings from recent research and inquiry. *Journal of Nursing Management, 5*, pp. 43–50.

Folstein, M. and Folstein, S. (1975). Mini mental state. A practical method for grading the cognitive state of patients for the clinician. *Journal of Psychiatric Research*, 12(3), pp. 189–198.

Forrest, D. (1989). The experience of caring. *Journal of Advanced Nursing*, 14, pp. 815–823.

Fossbinder, D. (1994). Patient perceptions of nursing care. *Journal of Advanced Nursing*, 20, pp. 1085–1093.

Fraley, R. C. (2010). A brief overview of adult attachment theory and research. http://internal. psychology.illinois.edu/~rcfraley/attachment.htm.

Fraser, M. (1996). *Conceptual Nursing in Practice. A Research-Based Approach* (2nd edn). London: Chapman and Hall.

Friedman, M. and Rosenman, R. (1974). *Type A Behaviour and Your Heart*. New York: Harper Row.

Gardner, R. (1992). Psychological care of neuro-oncology patients and their families. *British Journal of Nursing*, 11(11), pp. 553–556.

Gaut, D. (1983). Development of a theoretically adequate description of caring. *Western Journal of Nursing Research*, 5(4), pp. 313–324.

George, J. B. (2002). *Nursing Theories. The Base For Professional Nursing Practice* (5th edn). Upper Sadler River, NJ: Prentice Hall.

Gessler, S., Low, J., Daniells, E., Williams, R., Brough, V., Tookman, A., and Jones, L. (2008). Screening for distress in cancer patients: is the distress thermometer a valid measure in the UK and does it measure change over time? A prospective validation study. *Psycho-oncology* 17(6), pp. 538–547.

Gibbs, G. (1988). *Learning by Doing. A Guide to Teaching and Learning Methods*. Oxford Polytechnic: Further Education Unit.

Gibbs, M. and Priest, H. (2009). Exploring the physical health needs of people with learning disabilities: facilitating student engagement in learning, using Kolb's experiential learning cycle. *Nurse Education in Practice*. (online version, published 23 May 2009, DOI:10.1016/j.nepr.2009.04. 005).

Gilbert, J. G. and Weitz, R. D. (1949). *Psychology for the Profession of Nursing*. New York: Ronald Press.

Girot, E. (1991). Sociology and psychology in nursing. *Senior Nurse*, 11(2), pp. 5–8.

GNC (1952). *Syllabus of Subjects for Examination for the Certificate of General Nursing.* London: General Nursing Council for England and Wales.

GNC (1962). *Syllabus of Subjects for Examination for the Certificate of General Nursing.* London: General Nursing Council for England and Wales.

Goldberg, D., Huxley, P. (1980). *Mental Illness in the Community. The Pathway to Psychiatric Care.* London: Tavistock Publications.

Golding, K. S. (2007). Nurturing Attachments: Supporting Children Who Are Fostered or Adopted. London: Jessica Kingsley Publishers.

Greenwood, J., and King, M. (1995). Some surprising similarities in the clinical reasoning of 'expert' and 'novice' orthopaedic nurses: report of a study using verbal protocols and protocol analyses. *Journal of Advanced Nursing*, 22, pp. 907–913.

Griffin, A. (1983). A philosophical analysis of caring in nursing. *Journal of Advanced Nursing*, 8, pp. 289–295.

Grigsby, K. A. and Megel, M. E. (1995). Caring experiences of nurse educators. *Journal of Nursing Education*, 34(9), pp. 411–418.

Gross, R. and Kinnison, N. (2007). *Psychology for Nurses and Allied Health Professionals: Applying Theory to Practice.* London: Hodder Education.

Hallett, R. (1991). Psychological preparation for surgery: a critical analysis. *Clinical Psychology Forum*, February 1991, pp. 20–24.

Hamilton, M. (1959). The assessment of anxiety states by rating. *British Journal of Medical Psychology*, 32, pp. 50–55.

Hanson, L. E., and Smith, M. J. (1996). Nursing students' perspectives: experiences of caring and not-so-caring interactions with faculty. *Journal of Nursing Education*, 35(3), pp.105–112.

Hargie, O. (2010). *Skilled Interpersonal Communication: Research, Theory and Practice* (5th edn). London: Routledge.

Harlow, H. (1958). The nature of love. *American Psychologist*, 13, pp. 573–685 (http://psychclassics. yorku.ca/Harlow/love.htm).

Harrison, A. (2001). The mental health needs of patients in physical care settings. *Nursing Standard*, 15(51), pp. 47–54.

Hawkins, J., and Hollinworth, H. (2003). Living theory: enhancing the psychological support of patients. *British Journal of Nursing*, 12(9), pp. 543–548.

Hayes, N. (1994). *Foundations of Psychology.* London: Routledge.

Hayward, J. (1975). *Information: A Prescription Against Pain.* London: Royal College of Nursing.

Heath, H. and Freshwater, D. (2000). Clinical supervision as an emancipatory process: avoiding inappropriate intent. *Journal of Advanced Nursing*, 32(5), pp. 1298–1306.

Heider, F. (1958). *The Psychology of Interpersonal Relations.* New York: Wiley.

Henderson, S. (2002). Factors impacting on nurses' transference of theoretical knowledge of holistic care into clinical practise. *Nurse Education in Practice 2*, pp. 244–250.

Holmes, T. H. and Rahe, R. H. (1967). The social readjustment rating scale. *Journal of Psychosomatic Research*, 11(2), pp. 213–218.

Holyoake, D. (1997). Exploring the nature of nurse interaction using an interaction interview schedule: the results. *Psychiatric Care* 4, pp. 83–87.

Hochschild, A. (1983). *The Managed Heart: Commercialization of Human Feeling.* Berkeley: University of California Press.

Hoyt, M. (1995). *Brief Therapy and Managed Care: Readings for Contemporary Practice.* San Francisco: Jossey-Bass.

Hyland, M., and Donaldson, M. (1989). *Psychological Care In Nursing Practice.* London: Scutari Press.

James, N. (1989). Emotional labour: skill and work in the social regulation of feeling. *Sociological Review*, 37, pp. 15–42.

James, N. (1992). Care = organisation + physical labour + emotional labour. *Sociology of Health and Illness*, 14(4), pp. 488–509.

James, W. (1890). *Principles of Psychology.* New York: Holt and Co.

Jarrett, N. and Payne, S. (1995). A selective review of the literature on nurse–patient communication: has the patient's contribution been neglected? *Journal of Advanced Nursing*, 22, pp. 72–78.

Jeffery, R. (1979). Normal rubbish: deviant patients in casualty departments. *Sociology of Health and Illness* 1(1), pp. 90–107. (online version, published 28 June 2008, DOI: 10.1111/1467-9566. ep11006793).

Johnson, M. (1982). Recognition of patients' worries by nurses and by other patients. *British Journal of Clinical Psychology*, 21, pp. 255–261.

Johnson, M. and Webb, C. (1995). Rediscovering unpopular patients: the concept of social judgement. *Journal of Advanced Nursing*, 21 (3), pp. 466–475.

Johnstone, L. and Dallos, R. (2006). Introduction to formulation. In L. Johnstone and R. Dallos (Eds), *Formulation in Psychology and Psychotherapy. Making Sense of People's Problems* (pp. 1–16). Hove: Routledge.

Jones, A. C. (2005). Transference, counter-transference and repetition: some implications for nursing practice. *Journal of Clinical Nursing*, 14(10), pp. 1177–1184.

Jost, K. E. (1995). Psychosocial care: document it. *American Journal of Nursing*, July 1995, pp. 46–49.

Kagan, C., and Evans, J. (1998). *Professional Interpersonal Skills for Nurses* (2nd edn). Cheltenham: Nelson Thornes.

Kelly, G. (1955, reprinted 1990). *The Psychology of Personal Constructs*. London: Routledge.

Kelly, M. and May, D. (1982). Good and bad patients: a review of the literature and a theoretical critique. *Journal of Advanced Nursing*, 7(2), pp. 147–156.

Kent, G., Wills, G., Faulkner, A., Parry, G., Whipps, M., and Coleman, R. (1996). Patient reactions to met and unmet psychological need: a critical incident analysis. *Patient Education and Counselling*, 28(2), pp. 187–190.

King, L. and Appleton, J. (1997). Intuition: a critical review of the research and rhetoric. *Journal of Advanced Nursing*, 26, pp. 194–202.

Kirschenbaum, H. and Henderson, V. (1990). *The Carl Rogers Reader*. London: Constable.

Kitson, A. (1993). Formalising concepts related to nursing and caring. In A. Kitson (Ed.), *Nursing: Art and Science* (pp. 25–47). London: Chapman and Hall.

Kitson, A. (2003). A comparative analysis of lay-caring and professional (nursing) caring relationships. *International Journal of Nursing Studies*, 40, pp. 503–510.

Kitwood, T. (1997). *Dementia Reconsidered. The Person Comes First*. Buckingham: Open University Press.

Kolb, D. A. (1984). *Experiential Learning: Experience as the Source of Learning and Development*. Englewood Cliffs: Prentice Hall.

Koldjeski, D. (1990). Toward a theory of professional nursing caring: a unifying perspective. In M. Leininger, and J. Watson (Eds), *The Caring Imperative in Education* (pp. 45–57). New York: National League for Nursing.

Kunyk, D. and Olson, J. (2000). Clarification of conceptualizations of empathy. *Journal of Advanced Nursing*, 35(3), pp. 317–325.

Kyle, T. V. (1995). The concept of caring: a review of the literature. *Journal of Advanced Nursing*, 21, 506–514.

Larson, D. (1987). Comparison of cancer patients' and professional nurses' perceptions of important nurse caring behaviors. *Heart and Lung*, 16(2), pp. 187–193.

Lawton, M., van Haitsma, K, and Klapper, J. (1999). Observed emotion rating scale (OERS). http:// www.abramsoncenter.org/pri/documents/observedemotion.pdf.

Lea, A. and Watson, R. (1996). Caring research and concepts: a selected review of the literature. *Journal of Clinical Nursing*, 5, pp. 71–77.

Lea, A., Watson, R. and Deary, I. (1998). Caring in nursing: a multivariate analysis. *Journal of Advanced Nursing*, 28(3), pp. 662–671.

Ley, P. (1988). *Communicating with Patients.* London: Chapman and Hall.

Leininger, M. (1981). The phenomenon of caring: importance, research questions and theoretical considerations. In M. Leininger (Ed.), *Caring: An Essential Human Need. Proceedings of Three National Caring Conferences* (pp. 3–15). Thorofare, NJ: Charles B. Slack.

Linden, W. (1996). Psychosocial interventions for patients with coronary artery disease. A meta-analysis. *Archives of Internal Medicine*, 156, pp. 745–753.

Loftus, E. F. and Palmer, J. C. (1974). Reconstruction of auto-mobile destruction: an example of the interaction between language and memory. *Journal of Verbal Learning and Verbal Behaviour*, 13, pp. 585–589.

London School of Economics (LSE) (2006). *The Depression Report. A New Deal for Depression and Anxiety Disorders.* London: Centre for Economic Performance's Mental Health Policy Group, LSE.

Low, C., Beran, T. and Stanton, A. (2007). Adaptation in the face of advanced cancer. In M. Feuerstein (Ed.). *Handbook of Cancer Survivorship* (pp. 211–228). New York: Springer.

Luft, J. and Ingham, H. (1955). The Johari window, a graphic model of interpersonal awareness. Proceedings of the Western Training Laboratory in Group Development. Los Angeles: UCLA.

Lugton, J. and McIntyre, R. (Eds) (2005). *Palliative Care. The Nursing Role* (2nd edn). Edinburgh: Elsevier.

MacLeod, M. (1994). 'It's the little things that count': the hidden complexity of everyday clinical nursing practice. *Journal of Clinical Nursing*, 3, 6, pp. 361–368.

McCabe, C. and Timmins, F. (2006). *Communication Skills for Nursing Practice*. Basingstoke: Palgrave Macmillan.

McCance, T. V., McKenna, H. P. and Boore, J. (1997). Caring: dealing with a difficult concept. *International Journal of Nursing Studies*, 34(4), pp. 241–248.

McCrae, R. R. and Costa, Jr., P. T. (1987). Validation of the five-factor model of personality across instruments and observers. *Journal of Personality and Social Psychology*, 52, pp. 81–90.

McGee, P. (2005). *Principles of Caring*. Cheltenham: Nelson Thornes.

McGhie, A. (1979). *Psychology as Applied to Nursing* (7th edn). Edinburgh: Churchill Livingstone.

McKenzie, N. (1951). *Aids to Psychology for Nurses*. London: Ballière Tindall.

McMahon, R. (1991). Therapeutic nursing: theory, issues and practice. In R. McMahon and A. Pearson (Eds), *Nursing as Therapy* (pp. 1–25). London: Chapman and Hall.

Marriner Tomey, A. (1998). The elements of nursing: a model of nursing based on a model of living. In A. Marriner Tomey and M. R. Alligood (Eds), *Nursing Theorists and Their Work* (4th edn) (pp. 321–332). St. Louis: Mosby.

Maslow, A. (1954). *Motivation and Personality*. New York: Harper and Row.

Maslow, A. (1973). *The Farther Reaches of Human Nature*. Harmondsworth: Penguin.

Mayeroff, M. (1971). *On Caring*. New York: Harper and Row.

Menzies Lyth, I. (1960). Social systems as a defence against anxiety. *Human Relations*, 13, pp. 95–121. http://www.moderntimesworkplace.com/archives/ericsess/sessvol1/Lythp439.opd.pdf.

Miller, S. M. (1987). Monitoring and blunting: validation of a questionnaire to assess styles of information seeking under threat. *Journal of Personality and Social Psychology*, 52, pp. 345–353.

MIND (2010) Statistics 1: how common is mental distress? http://www.mind.org.uk/help/research_and_policy/statistics_1_how_common_is_mental_distress#depression.

Mitchell, M. (1994). Preoperative and postoperative psychological nursing care. *Surgical Nurse*, 7(3), pp. 22–25.

Mitchell, M. (1997). Patients' perceptions of pre-operative preparation for day surgery. *Journal of Advanced Nursing*, 26(2), pp. 356–363.

Mitchell, M. (2002). Guidance for the psychological care of day case surgery patients. *Nursing Standard*, 16(40), pp. 41–43.

Mitchell, M. (2005). *Anxiety Management in Adult Day Surgery: A Nursing Perspective*. London: Whurr.

Moccia, P. (1990). Deciding to care: a way to knowledge. In M. Leininger and J. Watson (Eds), *The Caring Imperative in Education* (pp. 207–215). New York: National League for Nursing.

Morris, J., Goddard, M., and Roger, D. (1989). *The Benefits of Providing Information to Patients*. York: Centre for Health Economics.

Morrison, P. (1991). The caring attitude in nursing practice: a repertory grid study of trained nurses' perceptions. *Nurse Education Today*, 11, pp. 3–12.

Morrison, P. (1993). Teaching psychology: the Australian view. *Nursing Standard*, 7(44), pp. 25–27.

Morrison, P. and Burnard, P. (1997a). *Caring and Communicating. The Interpersonal Relationship in Nursing* (2nd edn). Basingstoke: Macmillan.

Morrison, P. and Burnard, P. (1997b). *Caring and Communicating. Facilitators' Manual.* Basingstoke: Macmillan.

Morse, J. M. (1991). Negotiating commitment and involvement in the nurse–patient relationship. *Journal of Advanced Nursing*, 16, pp. 455–568.

Morse, J. M., Solberg, S. M., Neander, W. L, Bottorff, J. L. and Johnson, J. L. (1990). Concepts of caring and caring as a concept. *Advances in Nursing Science*, 13(1), pp. 1–14.

Muxlow, J. (1995). The relationship between nurse and patient. *Professional Nurse*, 11(1), pp. 63–65.

National Archives (1990). National Health Service and Community Care Act 1990. http://www. legislation.gov.uk/ukpga/1990/19/contents.

NHS (2007). Cancer Reform Strategy . http://www.cancer.nhs.uk/documents/cancer_reform_strategy/ cancer_reform_strategy.pdf.

NHS (2009). About the NHS. http://www.nhs.uk/NHSEngland/thenhs/about/Pages/overview.aspx.

NHS (2010). Choice in the NHS. http://www.nhs.uk/CHOICEINTHENHS/Pages/Choicehome. aspx.

NHS Choices (2010). National Service Frameworks. http://www.nhs.uk/nhsengland/NSF/pages/ Nationalserviceframeworks.aspx.

NICE (2002). Improving outcomes in breast cancer. http://www.nice.org.uk/nicemedia/live/10887/ 28763/28763.pdf.

NICE (2004a). Anxiety. Management of anxiety in adults in primary, secondary and community care. http://guidance.nice.org.uk/CG22/Guidance/pdf/English.

NICE (2004b). *Improving Supportive and Palliative Care for Adults with Cancer.* London: NICE.

NICE (2005). Post-traumatic stress disorder (PTSD): the treatment of PTSD in adults and children. http://www.nice.org.uk/nicemedia/pdf/CG026publicinfo.pdf.

NICE (2009). Depression in adults (update). http://www.nice.org.uk/nicemedia/pdf/Depression_ Update_FULL_GUIDELINE.pdf.

NICE (2010). Chest pain of rrecent onset. http://guidance.nice.org.uk/CG95/NICEGuidance/pdf/ English.

NICE (2011). Cash boost for psychological therapies to treat mental health. http://www.nice.org.uk/.

Nichols, K. A. (1985). Psychological care by nurses, paramedical and medical staff: essential developments for the general hospitals. *British Journal of Medical Psychology*, 58, pp. 231–240.

Nichols, K. (1993). *Psychological Care in Physical Illness* (2nd edn)*.* London: Chapman and Hall.

Nichols, K . (2003). *Psychological Care for Ill and Injured People.* Maidenhead: Open University Press.

Nichols, K. (2005). Why is psychology still failing the average patient? *The Psychologist*, 18(1), pp. 26–27.

Nightingale, F. (1859, reprinted 1980). *Notes on Nursing. What It Is and What It Is Not.* Edinburgh: Churchill Livingstone.

Niven, N. (2006). *The Psychology of Nursing Care* (2nd edn). Basingstoke: Palgrave Macmillan.

NMC (2004). *Professional Conduct: Standards for Conduct, Performance and Ethics.* London: Nursing and Midwifery Council.

NMC (2007). Supporting direct care through simulated practice learning in the pre-registration nursing programme. http://www.nmc–uk.org/Documents/Circulars/2007circulars/NMCcircular36_2007.pdf.

NMC (2010). *Pre-Registration Nursing Education in the UK.* London: Nursing and Midwifery Council. http://standards.nmc–uk.org/PreRegNursing/non–statutory/Pages/overview.aspx.

Nolan, M. (2000). Skills for the future. The humanity of caring. *Nursing Management*, 7(6), pp. 23–29.

Nolan, M., Keady, J. and Aveyard, B. (2001). Relationship centred care is the next logical step. *British Journal of Nursing*, 10(12), p. 757.

O'Connell, B. and Radloff, P. (1995). Is holism an appropriate philosophy for nursing? *Nursing Inquiry,* 2, 59.

Ogden, P. and Minton, K. (2006) *Trauma and the Body: A Sensorimotor Approach to Psychotherapy.* Norton.

Orem, D. (1995) *Nursing: Concepts for Practice* (5th edn). New York: McGraw Hill.

Paget, M. (2010). Developing relationships. In L. de Raeve, M. Rafferty and M. Paget, *Nurses and Their Patients: Informing Practice Through Psychodynamic Insights* (pp. 25–37). Keswick: M & K Publishing.

Paley, J. (2001). An archaeology of caring knowledge. *Journal of Advanced Nursing*, 36(2), pp. 188–198.

Pålsson, M.-B. E. and Norberg, A. (1995). Breast cancer patients' experiences of nursing care with the focus on emotional support: the implementation of a nursing intervention. *Journal of Advanced Nursing*, 21, pp. 277–285.

Parliamentary and Health Service Ombudsman (2010). Annual Reports. http://www.ombudsman.org.uk/about–us/publications/annual–reports.

Paulson, D. S. (2004). Taking care of patients and caring for patients are not the same. *AORN Journal*, 79, pp. 359–60.

Peacock, J. and Nolan, P. (2000). Care under threat in the modern world. *Journal of Advanced Nursing*, 32(5), pp. 1066–1070.

Pegram, A. (1992). How do qualified nurses perceive care? *Journal of Clinical Nursing*, 11, pp. 48–49.

Pepin, J. I. (1992). Family caring and caring in nursing. *Image. Journal of Nursing Scholarship*, 24(2), pp. 127–131.

Peplau, H. (1952). *Interpersonal Relations in Nursing*. New York: G. P. Putnam and Sons.

Phillips, P. (1993). A deconstruction of caring. *Journal of Advanced Nursing*, 18, pp. 1554–1558.

Phillips, K. D., Blue, C., Brubaker, K., Fine, M., Kirsch, M. J., Papazian, C., Reister, C. M. and Sobiech, M. (1998). Sister Callista Roy: adaptation model. In A. Marriner Tomey and M. R. Alligood (Eds), *Nursing Theorists and their Work* (4th edn) (pp. 243–266). St. Louis: Mosby.

Philpot, T. (2001). Clean, modern, inhuman. *Nursing Times*, 97(4), pp. 28–29.

Priest, H. (1999a). Psychological care in nursing education and practice: a search for definition and dimensions. *Nurse Education Today*, 19(1), pp. 71–78.

Priest, H. (1999b). Novice and expert perceptions of psychological care and the development of psychological care-giving abilities. *Nurse Education Today*, 19(7) pp. 556–563.

Priest, H.M. (2001). Psychological care in nursing: the public and the private face. Unpublished doctoral thesis, Keele University.

Priest, H. (2002). The phenomenology of psychological caregiving in nursing. *International Journal for Human Caring*, 6(3), pp. 8–14

Priest, H. (2006). Helping student nurses to identify and respond to the psychological needs of physically ill patients: implications for curriculum design. *Nurse Education Today*, 26, pp. 423–439.

Priest, H. (2010). Effective psychological care for physically ill patients in hospital. *Nursing Standard*, 24(44), pp. 48–56.

Radsma, J. (1994). Caring and nursing: a dilemma. *Journal of Advanced Nursing*, 20, pp. 444–449.

Ragins, M. (2002). Recovery with severe mental illness: changing from a medical model to a psychosocial rehabilitation model. http://www.village–isa.org/Ragin's%20Papers/recov.%20with %20severe%20MI.htm.

Ramirez, A. and House, A. (1998). Common mental health problems in hospital. In T. Davies and T. Craig (Eds) *ABC of Mental Health* (pp. 9–11). London: BMJ Books.

Ramprogus, V. (1995). *The Deconstruction of Nursing*. Aldershot: Avebury.

Read, S. and Morris, H. (2009). *Living and Dying with Dignity: The Best Practice Guide to End of Life Care for People with a Learning Disability*. London: Mencap.

Read, S. (2008). Loss, bereavement, counselling and support: an intellectual disability perspective. *Grief Matters*, 11(2), pp. 54–59.

Regel, S. and Rogers, D. (2002). *Mental Health Liaison: A Handbook for Health Care Professionals*. London: Ballière Tindall.

Reynard, C., Reynolds, J., Watson, B., Mathews, D., Gibson, L. and Clarke C. (2007). Understanding distress in people with severe communication difficulties: developing and assessing the disability distress assessment tool (DisDAT). *Journal of Intellectual Disability Research*, 51(4), p. 277.

Reynolds, W. and Scott, B. (2000). Do nurses and other professional helpers normally display much empathy? *Journal of Advanced Nursing*, 31(1) pp. 226–234.

Rimon, D. (1979). Nurses' perception of their psychological role in treating rehabilitation patients: a study employing the Critical Incident Technique. *Journal of Advanced Nursing*, 4, pp. 403–413.

Robertson, J. and Robertson, J. (1989). *Separation and the Very Young*. London: Free Association Books.

Rogers, C. (1957). The necessary and sufficient conditions of therapeutic personality change. In H. Kirschenbaum and V. Henderson (1990). *The Carl Rogers Reader* (pp. 219–235). London: Constable.

Rogers, C. (1958). The characteristics of a helping relationship. In H. Kirschenbaum and V. Henderson (1990). *The Carl Rogers Reader* (pp. 108–126). London: Constable.

Rogers, C. (1970). *On Becoming a Person: A Therapist's View of Psychotherapy*. Boston: Houghton Mifflin.

Roper, N., Logan, W. and Tierney A. (1980). *The Elements of Nursing*. Edinburgh: Churchill Livingstone.

Ross, F. (2010). Poor organisational cultures erode compassionate care. http://www.nursingtimes.net/5018269.article.

Ross, L. (1977). The intuitive psychologist and his shortcomings: distortions in the attribution process. In L. Berkowitz (Ed.), *Advances in Experimental Social Psychology* (vol. 10). New York: Academic Press.

Rotter, J. (1966). Generalised expectancies for internal *vs* external control of reinforcement. *Psychological Monographs*, 80(1), pp. 1–26.

Roy, C. (1980). *Introduction to Nursing: An Adaptation Model*. Englewood Cliffs: Prentice-Hall.

Royal College of Nursing (1992). *The Value of Nursing*. London: Royal College of Nursing.

Royal College of Nursing (2004). *Quality Education for Quality Care: Priorities and Actions*. London: Royal College of Nursing.

Royal College of Nursing (2008). Report on a scoping exercise to identify priority topics for national audit on the essence of care. http://www.rcn.org.uk/__data/assets/pdf_file/0008/250964/FINAL REPORTONSCOPINGEXERCISEONNATIONALAUDITOFESSENCEOFCARE_2.pdf.

Royal College of Nursing (2009). *Clinical Governance*. London: Royal College of Nursing. http://www.rcn.org.uk/development/practice/clinical_governance.

Royal College of Nursing (2011). NHS reforms must not threaten improvements. http://www.rcn.org.uk/newsevents/news/article/uk/nhs_reforms_must_not_threaten_improvements.

Rytterström, P., Cedersund, E. and Arman, M. (2009). Care and caring culture as experienced by nurses working in different care environments: a phenomenological-hermeneutic study. *International Journal of Nursing Studies*, 46, pp. 689–698.

Sadler, J. J. (1997). Defining professional nurse caring: A triangulated study. *International Journal for Human Caring*, 1(3), pp. 12–21.

Sage, N., Sowden, M., Chorlton, E. and Edeleanu, A. (2008). *CBT for Chronic Illness and Palliative Care: A Workbook and Toolkit*. Chichester: John Wiley and Sons Ltd.

Salvage, J. (1990). Theory and practice of 'the new nursing'. *Nursing Times*, 86(4), pp. 42–46.

Sarafino, E. (2005). *Health Psychology: Bio-psychosocial Interactions* (5th edn). Chichester: Wiley.

Saywell, E. (1924). *Sidelights from the New Psychology: A Handbook for Nurses*. London: The Scientific Press.

Schön, D. (1991). *The Reflective Practitioner* (2nd edn). San Francisco: Jossey Bass.

Seligman, M. E. P. (1975). *Helplessness: On Depression, Development, and Death*. San Francisco: W.H. Freeman.

Selyé, H. (1956). *The Stress of Life*. New York: McGraw-Hill.

Sheldon, L. K. (2007). Communication in oncology care: the effectiveness of skills training workshops for healthcare providers. *Clinical Journal of Oncology Nursing*, 9 (3), pp. 305–312.

Smith, P. and Gray, B. (2001). Emotional labour of nursing revisited: caring and learning 2000. *Nurse Education in Practice*, 1, pp. 42–49.

Sourial, S. (1997). An analysis of caring. *Journal of Advanced Nursing*, 26, pp. 1189–1192.

Staden, H. (1998) Alertness to the needs of others: a study of the emotional labour of caring. *Journal of Advanced Nursing*, 27, pp. 147–156.

Stockwell, F. (1984). *The Unpopular Patient*. London: Royal College of Nursing.

Sully, P. and Dallas, J. (2005). *Essential Communication Skills for Nursing*. Edinburgh: Elsevier Mosby.

Swanwick, M. and Barlow, S. (1994). How should we define the caring role? Broadening the parameters of the concept of care. *Professional Nurse*, May, pp. 554–559.

Tanner, C. A., Benner, P., Chesla, C. and Gordon, D. R. (1993). The phenomenology of knowing the patient. *Image. Journal of Nursing Scholarship*, *25*(4), pp. 273–280.

Taylor, B. J. (2005). *Reflective Practice. A Guide for Nurses and Midwives* (2nd edn). Buckingham: Open University Press.

Taylor, S. E. (1983). Adjustment to threatening events: a theory of cognitive adaptation. *American Psychologist*, 38(11), pp. 1161–1173.

Temoshok, L. (1987). Personality, coping style, emotions and cancer: towards an integrative model. *Cancer Surveys*, 6, pp. 545–567 (Supp).

The Centre for Economic Performance's Mental Health Policy Group (2006). The depression report: a new deal for depression and anxiety disorders (Layard Report). http://cep.lse.ac.uk/textonly/research/mentalhealth/DEPRESSION_REPORT_LAYARD.pdf.

Todd, S. (2006). A troubled past and present: a history of death and disability. In S. Read (Ed.), *Palliative Care in Learning Disability* (pp. 13–25). London: Quay Books.

Upton, D. (2009). *Introducing Psychology for Nurses and Healthcare Professionals*. Harlow: Pearson Educational.

UKCC (1989). *Project 2000 Rules. Circular PS&D/89/04(C)*. London: United Kingdom Central Council for Nursing, Midwifery and Health Visiting.

Victor, C. (2010). *Ageing, Health and Care*. University of Bristol: Policy Press.

Walker, J., Payne, S., Smith, P. and Jarrett, N. (2007). *Psychology for Nurses and the Caring Professions* (3rd edn). Maidenhead: Open University Press.

Warelow, P. (1996). Is caring the ethical ideal? *Journal of Advanced Nursing*, 24, pp. 655–661.

Watson, J. (1979). *Nursing: The Philosophy and Science of Caring*. Boston: Little, Brown.

Watson, J. (1988). *Nursing: Human Science and Human Care. A Theory of Nursing* (2nd edn). New York: National League for Nursing.

Watson, M. (1994). Psychological care for cancer patients and their families. *Journal of Mental Health*, 3(4), pp. 457–465.

Watson, J. (1999). *Post-modern Nursing and Beyond*. Edinburgh: Churchill Livingstone.

Watson, R. and Lea, A. (1997). The caring dimensions inventory (CDI): content validity, reliability and scaling. *Journal of Advanced Nursing*, 23, pp. 960–968.

Webster, R. (1991). Nurse education: behavioural and social sciences. *Senior Nurse*, 11(3), pp. 9–10.

Weiss, D. S. and Marmar, C. R. (1996). The impact of events scale-revised. In J. Wilson and T. M. Keane (Eds), *Assessing Psychological Trauma and PTSD* (pp. 399–411). New York: Guilford.

Wells, J. C. A. (1983). Critique of 'Psychology and nursing: The case for an empirical approach' by Lesley Wattley and Dave J. Müller. *Journal of Advanced Nursing*, 8, pp. 339–341.

Wertheimer, M. (1979). *A Brief History of Psychology* (2nd edn). New York: Holt, Rinehart and Winston.

WHO (1946). Constitution of the World Health Organization. http://www.who.int/governance/eb/who_constitution_en.pdf.

Wilkinson, J. (1996). All a matter of common sense? An introduction to psychology. *British Journal of Nursing*, 5(13), pp. 794–796, 809.

Wilson, I. (1931). *Psychology in General Nursing*. London: Edward Arnold.

Wilson-Barnett, J. (1976). Patients' emotional reactions to hospitalization: an exploratory study. *Journal of Advanced Nursing*, 1, pp. 351–358.

Wilson-Barnett, J. (1981). Keeping patients informed. *Nursing*, 31, pp. 1357–1358.

Wilson-Barnett, J. (1983). Critique of 'Psychology and nursing: The case for an empirical approach' by Lesley Wattley and Dave J. Müller. A question of choice. *Journal of Advanced Nursing*, 8, pp. 335–336.

Wilson-Barnett, J. (1988). Patient teaching or patient counselling? *Journal of Advanced Nursing*, 13, pp. 215–222.

Wilson-Barnett, J. (1994). Preparing patients for invasive medical and surgical procedures 3: Policy implications for implementing specific psychological interventions. *Behavioural Medicine*, 20, pp. 23–26.

Wondrak, R. (1998). *Interpersonal Skills for Nurses and Health Care Professionals*. Oxford: Blackwell Science.

Yerkes, R. M. and Dodson, J. D. (1908). The relation of strength of stimulus to rapidity of habit formation. *Journal of Comparative Neurology and Psychology*, 18(5), pp. 459–482.

Zigmond, A. S. and Snaith, R. P. (1983). The hospital anxiety and depression scale. *Acta Psychiatrica Scandinavica*, 67(6), pp. 361–370.

Index

Law, Ethics and Professional Issues for Nursing
A Reflective and Portfolio-Building Approach

By *Herman Wheeler*

This comprehensive new textbook covers core ethical and legal content for pre-registration nursing students. It provides readers with a sound understanding of the interrelationships between the NMC's code of conduct, standards and competencies, ethics and relevant sections of the English legal system.

The only truly integrated text in the field, it opens with overviews of law and nursing, and ethical theories and nursing. It goes on to explore key areas of contention – such as negligence, confidentiality and consent – from legal and ethical perspectives, mapping the discussion onto the NMC code of conduct. The chapters include objectives, patient-focused case scenarios, key points, activities, questions, areas for reflection, further reading and a summary. Case law and statutes and ethical theories are presented where appropriate.

Written by an experienced nurse-lecturer with a law and ethics teaching background, *Law, Ethics and Professional Issues for Nursing* is essential reading for all pre-registration nursing students, as well as students of other healthcare professions.

December 2011 | 360pp
Hb: 978-0-415-61888-5
Pb: 978-0-415-61889-2

For More Information
Please visit http://www.routledge.com/9780415618892

The Biological Basis of Mental Health Nursing

By *William T. Blows*

Written by an experienced nurse lecturer who also trained as a mental health nurse, this book explores the underlying biology associated with the pathology of mental health disorders and the related nervous system. Fully revised for this second edition, the text includes three new chapters on brain development, pharmacology and learning, behavioural and developmental disorders. Integrating up-to-date pharmacological and genetic knowledge with an understanding of environmental factors that impact on human biology, *The Biological Basis of Mental Health Nursing* covers topics including:

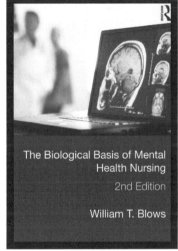

The Biological Basis of Mental Health Nursing

2nd Edition

William T. Blows

- the physiology of neurotransmission and receptors
- hormones and mental health
- the biology of emotions, stress, anxiety and phobic states
- the biology of substance abuse
- the pharmacology of psychoactive drugs
- developmental disorders
- brain anatomy and development
- the biology of behaviour
- genetics and mental health
- affective disorders: depression, mania and suicide
- schizophrenia
- autism and other syndromes
- the ageing brain and dementia
- degenerative diseases of the brain
- epilepsy.

December 2010: 246x174: 330pp
Hb: 978-0-415-56031-3
Pb: 978-0-415-57097-8

Accessibly laid out, with many of diagrams, tables and key points at the end of each chapter, this is an essential text for mental health nursing students, practitioners and educators.

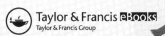
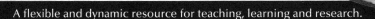